Never Giving Up
&
Never Wanting To

The Guide to Alzheimer's Care

Barry Tutor

Order this book online at www.trafford.com
or email orders@trafford.com

Most Trafford titles are also available at major online book retailers.

Printed in the United States of America.

ISBN: 978-1-4669-4880-8 (sc)
ISBN: 978-1-4669-4879-2 (hc)
ISBN: 978-1-4669-4878-5 (e)

Library of Congress Control Number: 2012917640

Trafford rev. 11/26/2013

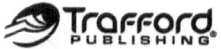 www.trafford.com

North America & international
toll-free: 1 888 232 4444 (USA & Canada)
fax: 812 355 4082

CONTENTS

For the millions of caregivers who serve in silence.

Preface

This book is not a theoretical text on caregiving, but is the journey I have taken with my wife and my mother as Alzheimer's disease (AD) has destroyed our lives. This book is also not an all-knowing, all-inclusive guide or owner's manual for caregiving; it is not even a step-by-step list of suggestions of how to care for your Alzheimer's patient. It is a bit of an autobiography mixed with many lessons learned and observations made by a solo caregiver. These are my bits and pieces of Alzheimer's information and stories I have gathered over the years while taking care of my mother and my wife through the various stages of this disease.

With not only being a solo caregiver, but also having to care for two Alzheimer's victims in two separate locations simultaneously, I had to develop a somewhat different approach to caregiving. While many have cared for two Alzheimer's victims, few nonprofessionals have done it simultaneously. And even fewer have had to care for a parent and a spouse simultaneously. To say I have had my hands full, even after my mother entered assisted living, is not an exaggeration for effect.

The information in this book comes from my far too many years of fighting the battles in the Alzheimer's war and watching others do the same. In my case, sometimes the battles were the same, just on two different fronts. Caring for two Alzheimer's patients simultaneously tends to give you double the experience in half the time.

We sit glued to our flat-screen televisions, watching people survive on islands, sing, dance, try to get lucky, lose weight, and race around the world. And they call this reality. You want reality—the type of "entertainment" that will never be on the television screen? Stop by a home that stars a life-altering or life-ending disease or condition, and meet the cast: one victim valiantly fighting a losing battle, a group of haggard caregivers, and a vast array of dwindling hopes and sincere prayers. This is reality, and for those who have not experienced this reality, the pages that follow will give you the reality of Alzheimer's Land. There is only one all-powerful, all-knowing judge in this reality show. And only He controls when you go home.

It is vitally important to prepare yourself for what's to come in your endeavor as an Alzheimer's caregiver. You will find out, hopefully not the hard way, that it is virtually impossible for a caregiver to have too much information or too many resources. It's a bit like having too much money. If you have too much money, you can always share it with those who are in need. If you have too many answers to the wide variety of Alzheimer's caregiving questions, you will be the first. So if you find yourself with all of the answers, share the information with the caregivers around you and the unfortunate caregivers coming behind you in this very crowded world of Alzheimer's.

I hope for three things to result from my book. First, I hope to show you that no matter how bad you have it, you are not alone in this journey—though it may seem like it more often than not. Remember, you do have the care recipient with you. At times, it may be of little solace, but at least you are not alone. Even though my wife, Lynne, is aphasic and seriously cognitively challenged, I still talk with her and make decisions after discussing options with her. So I am never really alone. Second, I hope you find a few places in my book to get a small laugh. If you are in it for the long haul, you certainly will need a laugh whenever you can find one. The laughs will certainly become harder to come by as the weeks turn into months and the months into years. My third hope is to never sell a copy of this book because the decades of research and clinical trials will finally bear fruit, and Alzheimer's will finally be cured.

I have tried to write this book like we are just two friends who now share a common bond of caring for Alzheimer's victims. In places, it may be preachy; other places may be vague. The preachiness comes from my passion about this disease and how it so indiscriminately destroys its victims and their families. The vagueness comes from how the disease affects each victim differently, and how each caregiver responds.

Our Fairy Tale

O nce upon a time, there lived in a tiny hamlet near the capital city of the United States a tall man and a beautiful lady. They were truly a wonderful couple who were so in love they could not imagine life without each other. They were nearly inseparable except for the occasional business journeys that the beautiful lady had to take. They were together for many, many years, having found adventures at home and even in faraway places like the land known as Vermont, where they spent many joyous vacations. They hoped to one day move to this magical land, where they would live out their lives together happily ever after.

Then one day, an all-knowing doctor with a big mustache told them they could not live out their lives together—whether in the tiny hamlet, beautiful Vermont, or any other wondrous place. The all-knowing doctor told the loving couple that the beautiful lady, whom so many adored, had a mysterious illness named Alzheimer's. With that devastating news, the wonderful couple knew that their fairy tale would come to an end, and their lives together and their plans would become distant memories that would eventually fade. They also knew that family and friends throughout the realm would come to their aid and make the premature departure of the beautiful lady easier for the tall man.

For some years, the beautiful lady had been troubled by things that caused her to visit a myriad of doctors. Doctors throughout the realm had tried, but alas had failed to discover what was troubling the beautiful lady. Then one day, the tall man and the beautiful lady visited the doctor with a big mustache who practiced in a nearby hamlet known as Reston. His citadel was across the trail from where the beautiful lady had worked years before in the field of undersea sailing vessels.

The tall man knew of this disease and what the future held for him and his family. Less than two years earlier, his mother, who had spent many years counseling military leaders in a strange place called the Pentagon, had developed the same disease. And it was by his hand—and only his hand—that his mother was cared for while still living in her humble cottage, which was also in the same tiny hamlet near the capital.

Acknowledgments

I thought long and hard about this book and its true meaning. I also put a lot of thought into these acknowledgments. This book may sound like sour grapes to some, but I know it represents the facts of life for many. No matter how long I stand watch over my wife and her battle with Early Onset Alzheimer's disease, I know that this battle is not only about the disease. If possible, it is more about the people who understand the necessity of individual compassion, dedication, love, and unwavering faith that make up the caregiving equation.

I acknowledge the people who understand the true meaning of answering the call to service on the personal level in often the most trying of circumstances. Specifically, the caregivers who have lived the nightmare of watching a loved one fighting a life-ending disease knowing that the only thing that can be done is tend to their loved ones' needs and pray their loved ones are in as little pain as possible until they hopefully, peacefully slip away.

I also recognize the people in our lives that have stood steadfast with us, answering our needs with thoughts, prayers, and deeds. Though some may deny their importance in our lives, for my mother and my wife, I thank from the bottom of our hearts: Linda "Shorty," Sharon, Mary, Amy, Marc, Rodney, Brigid, Linda, Ann, Stacy, Brooke, Billie, Andrea, Mez, and so many people whose names I have foolishly forgotten along the way who offered a bit of emotional support at the time I or we needed it. And a big group hug and thanks to the staff at Georgetown University Medical Center, Memory Disorders Program, and the staff and volunteers at Capital Caring.

I also want to thank radio personality Delilah, whose calming voice, words of love, and undeniable faith got me through many nights by reminding me to count my blessings for the many good years we had before the disease and for the ability to stand steadfastly by my loved ones when the disease took over.

I would be remiss if I did not acknowledge the people who just don't get it or the ones who got it and got the hell out of Dodge before the going got tough. The people who won't take a moment for a family member or friend who is facing a life-ending event are truly my heroes. Thanks for not cluttering up our lives and for shortening my Christmas card list.

Me—Caregiver

You may ask (and justifiably so), "Who are you to give me advice?" Me? I'm just another caregiver who hopes and prays that we will all gain some much-needed perspective on caring for someone with Alzheimer's disease and how it will rule and possibly ruin your life. And it will, in fact, rule your life. You will doubt decisions and spend time second-guessing yourself because you know that you can always do better. And what makes it worse is the person you are doing this for may not know you from Adam or Eve. To make things doubly worse, you have to do it all again tomorrow.

I have fought this battle every day without fail. I have fought on even though I have had so little sleep and several pains, ailments, and injuries. Forget the flu, the back strains, toothaches (including one from a tooth chipped by my wife's elbow), minor surgeries on my feet—and the list goes on. My mission is to care for the love of my life while forgetting or ignoring the physical pain that would put most on the sidelines, as it would me if I led a normal life.

My mother, Hazel, presented her early symptoms in 2002, and my wife, Lynne, presented in 2000 but was not diagnosed until 2006 at the age of fifty-eight. My caregiving knowledge and skills come from caring for the two most important people in my life. These skills also come from being involved with Alzheimer's support groups and observing at the Alzheimer's care facility that my mother entered in 2007 when I was no longer able to care for both singlehandedly, simultaneously, and at two locations. For over two and a half years, my mother lived in an Alzheimer's care facility that we called Happy Valley.

I feel the mission I was given—to care for two Alzheimer's patients—was given to me so I could provide them the best care possible and be their voice with the medical professionals while I could hopefully use my sense of humor to lift the spirits of my AD victims, family members, friends, and the people I have met along the way. And maybe I could also educate new caregivers and the uninformed about this disease and how it affects everybody. Then maybe it is also my mission to warn the uninformed that this disease is not just the disease of their parents and grandparents. It is also the disease of spouses, siblings, and children.

Through all the never-ending days, sleepless nights, and times of wondering what's next and how I am going to handle it, I have maintained my sense of humor. It helps me cope and often hides the pain of watching this slow-motion nightmare play itself out. It seems odd to still have a sense of humor, but little can be done to help the victim unless you can keep your head in the game and keep from upsetting the person you are caring for.

I find as I speak with people about caring for my two AD victims that maybe my assignment was not just random chance but guidance from a higher power. Many people will care for a parent or grandparent who suffers from Alzheimer's. It is more common than many think. But why did I get two? While you can do most anything with written instructions, you usually learn best with hands-on training. I am sure that the few years I cared for my mother comprised my apprenticeship, preparing me for the long haul of caring for my wife. Lessons learned while caring for my mother, watching the staff at the assisted living facility, attending support groups following my mother's diagnosis, and meeting other families experiencing Alzheimer's all had occurred before Lynne was diagnosed. When we finally got Lynne's diagnosis, I already had exposure, limited knowledge, and experience with the disease. So maybe the double dose of AD wasn't a curse but a blessing in disguise. And for some time, it was very well disguised!

Just who am I? Many times while dealing with this disease that has robbed me of my wife and my mother, I have asked myself the same question. I must tell you that I'm not a writer; I'm a storyteller. The wealth of experience I have with Alzheimer's care comes from caring for two drastically different Alzheimer's patients simultaneously.

Many have called me a hero, a good man, an expert, and even a saint. Many are amazed at my positive attitude, strength, and resilience in the face of such insurmountable odds. Others are surprised that I don't spend what little time I have available being mad at God for allowing such a disease to invade our home, the drug companies for not finding a cure, and the numerous doctors who failed to help us.

As I travel along the often rocky and always unpredictable path that is Alzheimer's care, I have found many people who want to know more about how to manage what some call the "long good-bye." Many have marveled that I have maintained a positive attitude and my sense of humor while many more wonder how I do what I do. But so many just want to know why I chose the role of solo caregiver. It's got to be more than love; it sure isn't for the glamour or the money. And it certainly is not for the challenge of seeing how long I will survive on too little sleep, too little exercise, and not always taking the best care of me.

Am I a control freak? Do things always have to be done my way? I answer a resounding yes to both questions, especially when it comes to Lynne's comfort and care. While the list of dementia and caregiving "experts" floating through my life grows, everyone has an opinion, a suggestion, or a thought on how I should handle our situation to take some of the pressure off myself. Most of their input is appreciated because it shows that at least some people have concerns for someone other than themselves. But as the disease continues, Lynne and her care are the most important things I have to be concerned with as long as she needs me. What's best for Lynne always takes precedence over my needs and my never-ending twenty-hour workdays.

Why do I spend twenty hours a day (on average) taking care of someone who has reached the stage of "I know you belong here, but who are you?" Yes, it breaks my heart to see my wife in this constant state of confusion punctuated by the very occasional spontaneous smile or laugh that always seems to come just at the right time but is gone as quickly as it came and may not return for days. These happy moments tell me that, at some level, she is still in there, and there is absolutely nothing I or anyone can do to bring her back. This is not only too bad for her, but also a tremendous loss for anyone who knows or knew her.

I have often been asked, "Why don't you get some help or just put her in a nursing home?" The answer is simple. When Lynne and I married, it was for the long haul—no matter what. You know the "richer, poorer, sickness, health" thing? We both took it seriously. So now that I am caring for her in what amounts to the twelfth year of her disease, I still maintain that as long as I am able to draw breath, I will care for her—whether she knows me or not. And I will never give up on her. It is possibly the ultimate demonstration of love—never giving up and never wanting to. It is not the jewelry, flowers, or expensive gifts on birthdays, anniversaries, and holidays that show how much we love. It is the sacrifices made when a terminal disease thrusts itself into a relationship.

My job is to care for Lynne, which means getting progressively less sleep. In year five, my typical night's sleep was about seven hours. As the years have gone by, I am now lucky to get four hours most nights and the occasional catnap, depending on Lynne's needs and her sleep patterns. Until October 2007, I also had my restless, often agitated early- and middle-stage AD mother two doors up the street. She thought nothing of calling at any hour of the day or night, having "heard something." This situation did not add to my sleep quantity or quality.

These numbers are just general estimates of how much sleep I manage to get, because there have been several nights that I have not slept at all because of Lynne's restlessness or her need to frequently use the bathroom. And while it is convenient to blame Lynne, my mother, and Alzheimer's for my sleep deprivation, I will admit that part of it is my fault. I am historically a light sleeper, and if I wake up during the night for any reason, I usually wake up so completely that it is difficult for me to go back to sleep. I don't recommend sleep deprivation week in and week out. So why don't I follow my own advice? I can sleep once my job of caring for Lynne is over.

I am also asked how I manage to stay awake and be functional twenty hours a day. I use no stay-awake drugs. I am caffeine-free and do not consume power bars or drinks. Since I am diabetic, I don't recharge with sugar. What is my explanation? Along with many other caregiving blessings, God has blessed me with the ability to function on little sleep, and He has given me the ability to go from zero to sixty the moment I wake.

As a solo caregiver, I am in caregiving mode twenty-four hours a day, seven days a week, 365 days a year. The role of solo caregiver is definitely not for everyone, and I highly discourage the practice if at all possible. What is my key to success? I sit as little as possible. When you sit, you relax, and sleep is just moments away. After surviving for years on so little sleep, you would be amazed how quickly those eyelids clamp shut when taking a moment for yourself. As a caregiver, there is almost always something to do that will keep you moving. If you run out of things to do, you are better at this caregiving thing than you give yourself credit for.

Something that surprised me as Lynne's disease progressed was that I have grown as a person, and I also feel that I have assumed some of my wife's personality since her decline began. I basically became both of us, because the strengths she brought into our relationship had to become my strengths also, or they would be lost. Throughout our relationship of over thirty-five years, we became essentially one person. Together, we make a great combination.

Something I noticed as the disease progressed was how I talk about Lynne and her condition. At first, I said, "My wife is ill" or "My wife is not feeling well." Then "ill" became "quite ill" or "very sick." I may have even used the word "dying" somewhere along the way.

Then one day, I said the word "terminal." As a layman, I have a strong knowledge base when it comes to Alzheimer's disease, and I can and do talk at length intelligently to anyone about the disease. I knew from the moment of diagnosis that living with Alzheimer's is a fatal, no-cure, no long-term planning, no golden years together scenario. The use of that word at that moment hit me; the woman I spent more than half my life with, adored, loved, and just always wanted to be with was going to be taken away from me little by little, brain cell by brain cell, until there would be nothing left but a hollowed-out shell of a person totally dependent on me every day for everything. This is when I finally understood the two rules of Alzheimer's disease. Rule one is that this disease is stealth, unrelenting, unforgiving, and uncaring; shows no mercy; maintains no age, sex, or race bias, and is irreversible. Rule two is that you can't change rule one, no matter how hard you try, no matter how hard you pray.

I want you to know my parents, Grady and Hazel Tutor. They were born and raised within a few miles of each other in Harnett County, North Carolina. They met and married in 1943 in Washington, DC, while he was stationed at Marine Corps Headquarters, Washington, and she was an Army civilian also working in Washington. I came along in 1952.

I introduce you to my father since he was unknowingly instrumental in how and why I care for others. He passed away in 1965 from a malignant brain tumor. My devoted mother was at his hospital bedside every day for nearly six months. With my father's passing, my mother fell into a deep depression that lasted for several years. At age twelve, since I was an only child, I was not only the man of the house, but I also pretty much had to grow up on my own. This situation gave me some perspective on how to deal with the problems that come with a family member with a terminal disease and its effects on the family.

When my father was diagnosed and hospitalized, his illness placed my mother in the position of being a single parent and a working mom. We were fortunate that back before the two-income family was commonplace, both of my parents had civilian positions with the US Army. My dad worked at Fort Myer in Arlington, Virginia, as a laundry and dry cleaning equipment mechanic, and my mother worked at the Pentagon as a computer systems analyst.

In my pre-caregiving days, I handled my mother's investments as well as ours, owned and operated two businesses, gardened, worked on our house as well as my mother's, and did the various chores inherent to homeownership and parenthood. This was frequently interrupted by one of our mothers needing help with something, needing a ride somewhere, or just needing someone to talk to because they were bored. Their close proximity made me the obvious target. Lynne's mother, Mary, lived with us, and my mother lived two houses up the street. Many times, usually in the middle of a project, I would hear the pitter-patter of little mother footsteps, which would always lead to, "I won't stop you, but I . . ." This, of course, always meant, *Stop everything, and pay attention to me.*

I certainly did not expect at any point in my life to get a free pass from God. So I just screw a smile on my face and just keep on going. I tell people I'm just like a duck. On the surface, you see a peaceful calm. But under the surface, what you don't see is the duck paddling like hell against the current so he won't be swept away.

I talk with God on a daily basis. The questions I ask are simple: Why us? Why Lynne at her young age? What can I do to better help Lynne and the others who are facing this turmoil? After years of asking, I have no better answer than to keep going, keep trying, and do your best. I also speak with God frequently about the lottery, and I'm still waiting for an answer on that.

I have tried not to embellish, exaggerate, or tell our story so that I always come out as the hero. Though many disagree; I am not the hero of this story. I am just a guy who fell in love with a petite brunette with a melt-your-heart smile and gorgeous blue eyes. Like my mother and the millions of other Alzheimer's victims, Lynne did not ask for this insidious disease. We have fought every symptom as long and as hard as we could, knowing we could not avoid the inevitable. And if you have not figured this out yet, I will continue to be at her side, helping her until God calls her home.

Many people have told me over the years that I needed to write this book. Some words of encouragement to help other caregivers in their daily battles in this seemingly never-ending war. After you read this, you will probably think, *I hope he is a better caregiver than he is a writer.* Trust me; I am.

Us Everlasting

Soul mates, split-aparts, twin souls, bashert, a match made in heaven, two peas in a pod, two halves of the same whole . . . and I am sure there are scores of other words and phrases used to describe the perfect relationship. While definitions, interpretations, and over analysis have, in some cases, muddied the meaning, Lynne and I truly feel that Richard Bach said it best: "No matter what else goes wrong around us, with that one person we're safe in our paradise. Our soul mate is someone who shares our deepest longings, our sense of direction. When we're two balloons, and together our direction is up, chances are we've found the right person. Our soul mate is the one who makes life come to life." Thomas Moore wrote, "A soul mate is someone to whom we feel profoundly connected, as though the communication and communing that take place between us were not the product of intentional efforts, but rather a divine grace. This kind of relationship is so important to the soul that many have said there is nothing more precious in life."

Lynne and I met in May 1976 shortly after my twenty-fourth birthday and shortly before her twenty-ninth. She had recently joined the company I had been working for since 1974. I was assigned to educate her on the work we did so she could develop quality control procedures and write a procedures manual for new employees. Much to the chagrin of my boss, we spent several hours nearly every day over the next few months working together so she would understand what we did to support the US Navy's Fleet Modernization Program. In all this time together, we became friends. We were just friends—not friends with benefits, just friends. We were only friends because we were married, but not to each other.

We met when my boss walked Lynne over to my desk, announced, "You work with him," and walked away. After I had found a chair for her, she sat down and confidently said, "Hi, my name is Lynne."

I responded with, "That should be easy to remember. My middle name is Len." With that, we discussed the variations of the name. Each day following, we sat and discussed the various parts of the work our group did for the Navy and chatted about our lives outside of the office. Our friendship grew quickly and continued to grow until Alzheimer's disease took over.

The company we worked for discouraged dating or marriage within the company, so once we had a relationship, it was kept totally out of the office. Though some suspected, there was never anything more than two coworkers occasionally going to lunch together. We managed to keep our relationship a secret, including our marriage, until I left the company for greener pastures in March 1983.

Since our relationship was a secret in the office and most of our friends worked with us, our wedding was just the two of us, our mothers, Lynne's two children, and a justice of the peace. We married outdoors on February 12, 1982, on the first overlook at Great Falls Park on the Virginia side of the Potomac River. We wanted to get married in the snow, but the Washington, DC-area is certainly not known for its snow, so we made do with what we had. But we did get our snow reward on our honeymoon weekend when we awoke to four inches of fresh snow in Williamsburg.

After we married, we still lived apart for over three months while the addition to the small house I lived in was being built. We changed my little three-bedroom, one-bath house into a six-bedroom, three-bath house so everyone would have space. Lynne, Mary, Nichole, and Mason moved in over Memorial Day weekend, and we finally started our lives together.

On the surface, we appear to be opposites. To be sure, no online dating service would ever have put us together. But over the decades together, we seldom argued and always made sure that the other one was happy with the decisions that affected both of us and our family.

I am truly at a loss for the words that would adequately describe our relationship—how much we loved and liked each other before the disease got in the way. We were best friends long before we were lovers, and possibly, if there is such a thing as past lives, best friends before. "I love you with every fiber of my being," "You complete me," and "I can't live without you" simply fail to convey the true depth of our relationship. Frankly, I am at a loss to convey to you how we were really just one person in two bodies. We were simply *us*—indivisible. This is why I relied on Messrs. Bach and Moore to do the heavy word lifting to start this chapter.

To say Lynne and I were in love is to understate the obvious. Our life together (until the Alzheimer's took us over) was truly an addiction—but in a very good way. Her strengths were my weaknesses, and vice versa. We rarely disagreed on anything and never really argued. Whenever we were together, we would always be touching and were often very playful. Many times, people commented on our holding hands and cutting up like we were dating or newlyweds. We simply could not get enough of each other. We talked about everything; we loved being together and hated when her job took her out of town, although her returns were always filled with great passion. We were joined at the heart, I guess you could say.

Lynne and I always talked about everything and held absolutely nothing back. We made our decisions together, planned and dreamed together, and quite often would discuss the events of the world and render comments accordingly. Even though now she is unable to speak more than a few garbled words and her decision-making skills have long since eroded, I still talk to her like nothing is wrong because that's the way we have always been. And I never ask if she understands because I know somewhere inside is the pre-Alzheimer's

Lynne who still understands and appreciates my input. I still value her opinion, even though she cannot render it except through a few facial expressions and the occasional chuckle, groan, or moan. If you are wondering if we talk about everything—I read every word of every draft of this book to her because it would not be real unless I did.

Lynne and I made love all the time—not physical, sexual lovemaking, but a mental, "I feel good because you feel good" type of thing. With both of us being only children, many are surprised that neither of us is the stereotypical selfish, me first brat. We each had the same goal in our relationship—making the other one happy.

Don't get me wrong; we did have a very physical, very active, very enjoyable sex life. We were like a couple of newlyweds on their honeymoon until the disease got in the way. When we were alone, we quite often took advantage of it. And we kept taking advantage until the disease got in the way in 2007.

Sex is an issue that may not affect your relationship when AD takes over your lives. Sex was never the key to our relationship. But we very willingly, joyously, and frequently participated in the physical aspect of our relationship. To it put more simply, we couldn't keep our hands off of each other and our clothes off the floor when we were alone.

In 1984, we had been married for a little more than two years when Lynne read an article about a survey regarding sex and second marriages. The article broke down age, frequency, and a variety of other elements. This article detailed how the longer a couple was together in a second marriage, the more the frequency due to factors not involving illness decreased. So on June 1, 1984, we started marking the calendar when we had sex. The practice continued until October 16, 2007, when the last mark was made on the calendar. The numbers stayed consistently high even though the Alzheimer's symptoms had really started showing themselves. And no, I did not keep the calendars for old time's sake. But I did keep a spreadsheet (no pun intended).

No, we were not sex addicts. We were addicted to each other and enjoyed a healthy, sometimes imaginative sex life until the morning of October 18, 2007. We were in the midst of having a roll in the hay when she looked at me like, *Who are you, and what are you doing?* That was the last time we attempted to have sex, though I did broach the subject a few times (after all, I am a guy), and while she does remember having sex, she really doesn't remember it was me who put a smile on her face for over thirty years while she put a smile on mine. In case you're wondering, we put 6,517 marks on the calendars.

You probably noticed I used the word "sex" instead of the phrase "making love." It is simply because we made love to each other every waking moment of every day we were together. Sex was just the physical expression of being together—and we certainly loved being together. The sixteen-inch height difference was no problem whatsoever!

One type of sex that seems to be popular among couples is makeup sex. We never had makeup sex in all the years we have been together. The reason is quite simple. We never really argued about anything. Sure, there were raised voices on occasion, but we are both rational, educated people, able to voice an opinion and listen to the opinions of others. So what's to argue about? I am here to tell you, in case you have not figured this out yet—life is far too short to waste your time arguing with the one you love. Yes, we would discuss our individual points of view, sometimes with raised voices, but would make rational decisions one way or the other or meet somewhere in the middle.

What was the key to our happiness? Aside from the generally agreeing on most everything, having similar goals, working in the same field, and the burning desire to always be together, we had one key ingredient that a lot of relationships struggle with—we were true equals in our partnership. We never competed against each other; we competed with each other. There was never a winner or a loser. We both won, because we were together, enjoying our time together.

Did we have and enjoy the perfect relationship? It wasn't perfect, but we came damn close. And if Alzheimer's disease had not taken over our lives, who knows what the future would have been like. Here is a strong piece of advice. Don't dwell on what-ifs. They do nothing but make you feel even worse—especially if the person you are caring for does not have the same regrets.

Lynne's Background

The most important person in my life is my wife, lover, partner in life, and most of all, my best friend. Lynne is the only child of Merle and Mary Goddard. Lynne was born in Oak Park, Illinois, in 1947. Before her sixth birthday, the little family relocated to Michigan. By the time Lynne left for college, because of her father's employment situation, she had moved more than a dozen times but never left the state of Michigan. In one move, they lived with relatives on a farm. Since the wife did not like having children in the house, Lynne was consigned to the screened porch to sleep. This probably was not the best arrangement for her since it was late fall when they arrived. Fortunately, they only lived there a few months.

In 1965, while attending Ferris State University, Lynne met Dale. They married in 1966 shortly after Lynne's nineteenth birthday. Soon after they married, Dale was drafted and eventually decided to make the Army his career. During the twelve-year marriage, they had two children—Nichole in 1970 and Mason in 1973. Lynne came to the Washington area in 1975 when Dale was transferred to the Pentagon. They separated in 1977 and divorced in 1978.

I am not here to tell Dale's and Merle's stories. Although they were good men, they have both passed away and are not really relevant to Lynne's story and my commitment to her and her care. But I felt you needed to know that Lynne, Nichole, and Mason were not immaculately conceived, hatched from an egg, or dropped off at the front door. (Although, as we move through this story, you will find the jury is still out on Mason and the latter.)

I often say that I wish you had known Lynne before the Alzheimer's silenced her generous, loving spirit. Lynne saw the good in everybody. She never met a person she did not like. That's not to say she did not have occasional disagreements with people, but her style was to always be low-key and non-confrontational. If she had difficulties with you, she would simply like you to death. Her goal was to make you uncomfortable by being so nice that you would feel like an ass for treating her badly.

Lynne loved people and seldom found or acknowledged anybody's flaws. She was blind to age, sex, and ethnicity. While she recognized a person's position in life, showing respect for his or her level of accomplishment, she treated each person like he or she was special. In Lynne's eyes, everybody was unique—but more importantly, no one was more unique than anybody else.

Before her vision became compromised, Lynne had been a voracious reader. When everyone was talking about the hot book, she was usually reading it. When Tom Clancy started looking for the *Red October*, Lynne was working as a government contractor for a US Navy submarine activity, so the book was required reading. When Harry Potter was the hot topic, she started reading the series. But her passion, pardon the pun, was romance novels, especially those of Johanna Lindsey. She read every one of them as soon as they hit the store shelf.

Through much of Lynne's career, she wrote and edited technical manuals for various government agencies. But she wished to become a children's author, so she took a course to learn the basics of children's writing and marketing. A few years before the disease started to become a problem, she did succeed in becoming a published children's author. Unfortunately, the disease once again got in the way of a dream.

In the 1990s, Lynne and I owned and operated a résumé writing service and small-business support office. During the day, I met with the clients and did the office part of the business while Lynne was working as a government contractor. Then at night, Lynne and I would write, edit, and type the jobs—sometimes well into the night.

The business was successful until the expenses of having the office ate up too much of the income and most everybody owned or had access to a computer.

As I face each day caring for my wife, I wonder what she's thinking. What makes her do or not do things, and does she still realize that she is terminally ill? In the early days, after she was finally diagnosed, she was still functioning—albeit at a reduced pace, but still functioning. She of course knew that she had Alzheimer's; there was no cure in sight, and the existing treatment would eventually become ineffective. We talked openly about the disease and how it would change her, how it would affect the family (especially me), and how the path yet to be traveled would become progressively more difficult. Since we already had some Alzheimer's experience with my mother's diagnosis sixteen months earlier, we had a good idea of what the future held. But what we did not realize at the time was that Alzheimer's disease affects different people in different ways and at different speeds.

Lynne's Alzheimer's

As the disease progresses, our days are still very ordinary, but the objective is still the same—take the best care of Lynne that I possibly am able to do. Along the way, I try to keep the house in decent shape; care for our pets, Dusty and Genie; and try to find a little time for me and my well-being.

I try my best to never say, "Do you remember?" "You probably don't remember . . ." "I'm sure you've forgotten . . ." or "I remember when you used to . . ." Why rub it in? I can tell by the look on her face that she knows she doesn't remember. I just try to phrase everything with enough information that I might fill in the ever-expanding gaps in her memory. Why should I remind both of us of what this disease did to our lives and the future we thought we had together?

For the most part, Lynne is stable enough when walking, so I don't have to confine her to the bed or a chair. When she walks through the room, I evaluate how stable she is and whether I have to physically direct her or keep her stable. As time marches on, even with her "geisha steps," I find myself walking with her more and more to make sure her face and the floor don't meet by accident. I also run interference with the sleeping dog or the cat that likes to play roadblock when you least expect. Even though Lynne does enjoy wandering around the house, she rarely attempts to open any closed door inside the house or attempt to leave the house without me escorting her.

When Lynne was still able to stay at home alone for a few hours while I visited my mother at Happy Valley, I would leave her a DVR full of reruns of various shows she enjoyed in the '70s and '80s. When she was bored with watching the television, she would sometimes do chores while I was gone just to help me out. This, of course, led to my having to redo many of these things after she went to bed. Sometimes I had to reload the dishwasher or put the clean dishes in the right cabinets or drawers. One day, she was nice enough to bag up the trash for the following day. That night, I had to retrieve the small trash can missing from the bathroom. But her heart was in the right place, and she was trying so desperately to fight the disease, so I never let on that she had done anything wrong.

Starting in year six and continuing for over two years, Lynne decided to simply lie in bed for twenty-three hours every day. She would get up to go to the bathroom and usually got up to eat. But then it was right back into bed. One day, she decided after lying in bed for over two years it was time to get up and tour the house, with occasional stops to play statue. I did not discourage the wandering; it was at least an improvement over vegetating—and after all, no matter how slight, it was exercise. I do intervene on occasion when she stands like a statue for fear she might doze off and fall. Now in year twelve, she spends much of her afternoon walking and playing statue for about an hour at a time.

This walking and wandering coincided with her starting to lounge on the love seat that she used as her chair. Every evening before the disease, she would curl up on this love seat while watching television or reading. She would quite often nap curled up on this love seat. When the Alzheimer's started getting worse, it appeared that she could not or would not get comfortable on her chair. She would sit upright, and no matter how often I told her she could sit back and relax, she would continue sitting like she was sitting on a straight-back chair. This lasted for a few years. Then one day, she sat on her little sofa, leaned back, put her feet up on the footstool, and within twenty minutes, she was sound asleep—just like she had done so many times before.

In year seven and continuing for approximately four years, it seemed Lynne had to urinate almost constantly. We went to her primary care physician to be sure that it was not a physical problem or a urinary tract infection. It appeared to simply be the progression of the disease. Her brain was sending signals that she had to urinate. Initially, on an average day, she would need to use the bathroom thirty to forty times a day. Nearly every trip was just a few drips because she was going so frequently. At one point, I began noting the times of our bathroom trips, thinking maybe I was exaggerating. For five days, I noted on a whiteboard in my office the times she went to the bathroom. In that five-day time span, her low number of trips was thirty-two in one day, and her high was forty-eight. One day, she went exactly every twenty minutes—just like clockwork—over a three-hour period. Fortunately, the ultrahigh frequency did subside after several months, but she still did have the urge more than fifteen times a day. Like everything else with this disease, things change—and sometimes they change for the better. After years of going and going, one day, she just started going a fairly normal number of times, urinating a fairly normal amount.

Among Lynne's many system failures, she has lost her ability to understand what she sees. It's not that she's going blind; her vision is still 20/20 with corrective lenses. Her brain is apparently not correctly processing the information. The best way to explain this is, of course, by example. You hear dogs barking, cats meowing, and birds singing. You can hear them perfectly well but cannot understand what they are saying, since you don't speak their languages. Fortunately, her vision difficulties are not so great that she has a problem navigating through doors, around furniture, and usually around the pets. Occasionally she does bump into the furniture or doorframes because of her lack of peripheral vision or because she's not paying full attention. Even her understanding of dark and light is sometimes affected to the point that she cannot tell if it's day or night.

Aphasia, a problem for victim and caregiver alike, destroys what little communication is necessary to express needs, discomfort, and emotions and just generally have a conversation. Lynne's aphasia has reached the point where she cannot express herself enough to tell me how she feels, what she wants or needs, or simply whether she's hungry, sleepy, bored, or needs to go to the bathroom. We have to depend on my perception of her facial expressions and body language to get things done when they need to be done. Her aphasia started with a simple stutter. I tell people that, before the disease, Lynne was a world-class talker to anybody about anything. Her aphasia was nearly undetectable when it first presented itself in 2000. She would speak well, as she always did, until she tried to say an alliterative phrase like "she sells seashells."

While she was still able to say short sentences or phrases with some clarity, she would consistently get lost in her sentence before she got to the subject. "I want . . ." or "I need . . ." certainly leaves the listener wanting more information, so they know what action to take if any action is required. As we entered year ten of the disease, Lynne's aphasia, coupled with some memory loss, had advanced to the point that her sentences became limited to only one or two garbled words. Her vocabulary has eroded to fewer than ten words. This is especially disturbing since Lynne spent many years writing and editing technical manuals for various government activities and documents for our small business and its clients. Words were her life.

No matter how many times I tell her that she can use a one-word subject like *pee, poop, bathroom, food, hungry, bed,* or whatever the subject, she has never been able to embrace this new concept because new concepts are new memories, and it's nearly impossible to implant a new memory—especially in the later stages of the disease. Even though she is "looking" for the action word in her mind, she is still thinking out the sentence in her mind and still getting lost in the middle of the sentence.

During a hospice recertification visit, the nurse practitioner asked, "Since Lynne is aphasic, how does she tell you what she needs?" It's very simple—based on years of verbal and nonverbal communication before the disease and in the early years of the disease; I can see it in her face and her body language. You pretty much develop a sense of what is needed, when it's needed, and why it's needed as you go through the various stages of the disease. It does not mean that you are always going to interpret the signals correctly, but when in doubt, it's best to err on the side of caution.

Before the disease took over, Lynne loved listening to music—especially the classic rock and roll of the '50s and '60s and country music. So I used music to help Lynne to relax and sleep. For several years, I would supply the type of music Lynne enjoyed to be played on a bedside CD player. Initially, the only music she truly enjoyed was by her all-time favorite, Elvis. So I focused on his soft rock, ballads, and gospel so the music would help her relax. Eventually, Elvis became less effective, so I started mixing in a few of her other favorite singers, which seemed to reestablish the CD player as a source of comfort. When she went to bed, I would load the CD player. Night after night for more than four years, Lynne listened to Elvis, Alan Jackson, George Strait, Reba McEntire, Alison Krauss, Emmylou Harris, and dozens more. Don't get me wrong; I love listening to music also, but it almost drove me nuts listening to the same songs hundreds of times until she no longer reaped the benefit from the CD player.

Unlike many dementia patients, including my mother, Lynne has seldom had any bouts of aggression or agitation and certainly no combativeness. I occasionally do get a pouty but stern "no," or sometimes she just ignores me, but that's about it. She occasionally will pull back when I reach to assist her in sitting, standing, or putting her feet on the bed. It may be that she does not see me or understand what I have said when I announce that I am going to assist her. I occasionally get a mild refusal of food or water, or she refuses to remain seated while I feed her, braid her hair, bathe her, or get her dressed. But thankfully, from the agitation standpoint, she is easy to care for in the grand scheme of things. I know many caregivers have it much worse, and some live in a constant state of fear, not knowing when or if their AD victim will become physically aggressive. All that being said Lynne still requires a 24/7 commitment from me and a lot of patience on my part.

Here's a fun little medical term—*myoclonic jerk*. Lynne's got it, and if you're in the late-onset crowd, you probably (if my sources are correct) will not have to worry about it. Myoclonic jerking is doctor-speak for the involuntary jerking of a muscle or muscle group. This jerking can happen infrequently or several times a minute. In Lynne's case, it is usually a frequent twitch or shake, but sometimes it escalates to where it looks like she is having a mild seizure. Fortunately, there is medication that calms Lynne's myoclonic jerking, and there are two schools of thought on its use. Ask your health care provider about medication, and discuss the pros and cons—just like everything else in the care of your AD victim—should you have issues with myoclonic jerking.

Whenever I dose Lynne for her myoclonic jerking, which varies from once every three weeks to once every two months, the following day, she has what I can only describe as a hangover that lasts approximately twenty-four hours. But the drug does lesson or stop the shaking temporarily. So I feel, as a quality-of-life issue, the drug is worth the price of a hangover.

When Lynne and I went to Georgetown during her second clinical trial, it was during the height of the cold and flu season. I had developed a mental checklist of places where we could come in contact with surfaces that may have cold or flu germs just waiting for an unsuspecting finger to transport them to a new home. I was diligent with every visit in ensuring that the germs stayed on the public surfaces and did not come home with us—except one day, I failed to sanitize my hands after all public contact ended. (The railing in the parking garage stairwell got me.) And of course, I brought home the flu bug, which certainly does put a cramp in caregiving. But it was worse when Lynne came down with the same flu.

The flu bug was less than kind to both of us, but especially to Lynne—probably because her immune system is compromised by the Alzheimer's and probably was additionally compromised by the clinical trial drug. Lynne's flu battle naturally included nausea, which of course provided us with a demonstration of memory issues when she had to vomit. We had issues on multiple fronts in dealing with the vomiting. It is something she clearly demonstrated she had forgotten. First, she had forgotten the warning signs and mechanics of vomiting. Second, she did not remember that she needed to be in a place suitable for vomiting, like in the bathroom or over any convenient trash can.

This was a crash course in caregiving as well as a logistics nightmare. It is also where I learned the value of having carpet cleaner and the large economy pack of paper towels. When Lynne needed to throw up the first time, she was standing in the middle of the bedroom. With no warning, she emptied her stomach. She was covered from chin to toe, and what was not stuck to her clothing lay in a puddle on the floor around her feet. This should summarize the necessity of keeping germs out of the caregiving facility.

But no good germ story would be complete without a follow-up germ story. After sorting through and putting enough of my mother's belongings into storage, we were able to free up one of our lost bedrooms. We decided, until Mom was moved back from Happy Valley, that we could use this bedroom as a guest room. So Lynne and I bought a new bedroom set, figuring we would eventually need a place for any live-in assistant to sleep anyway. We went to one of the local furniture stores to buy a new bedroom set for our rediscovered bedroom on the off chance we might have visitors who would want a place to sleep. When we arrived at the furniture store, the saleswoman, noting Lynne's very slow gait, offered a wheelchair, since we would likely be walking all over the store. We accepted the offer of the wheelchair, selected and purchased our furniture, and went home.

Over the next few days, Lynne presented a rash on her left forearm. I contacted hospice, and the nurse came out and examined Lynne's rash. It was a concern, especially since it had no apparent cause. The hospice nurse indicated that this rash may be a sign of many things— some of which sent a cold chill down my spine.

The following day, the rash was worse on her left arm and had presented on her right arm in approximately the same area. This is where I put two and two together and determined it was probably an allergic reaction to something on the wheelchair that we had used at the furniture store, since we had been no place else. A few days later, the rash was nothing but a memory—except it taught me a valuable lesson. Sanitize if you are using someone else's equipment, or just bring your own. Bringing your own is safer, and you won't be distracted from the loved one you are keeping safe while wiping down a wheelchair in the middle of a store.

Also, after an outing or a visitor coming into your home, remember to sanitize your AD victim's hands as well as your own. You don't know what they could have come in contact with while your back was turned. You need to also sanitize anything your guests may have touched, even if they appear to be in good health. It may look and sound like I am obsessed with germs, but my feeling is you cannot be too safe or too careful when it comes to your health and the health of your AD victim.

Lynne's Stories

When Lynne's mother, Mary, was sick, it dawned on me, because Lynne had never really had much of a reaction to reports of her mother's illness and probable demise, that maybe Lynne did not understand what was happening or whom it was happening to.

For as long as I knew Lynne's mother, she was known by three names: Mom, Grandma, and Mary. Toward the end of Mary's life, I was keeping Lynne up-to-date on her mother's decline. Lynne, for as long as I have known her, would cry at the drop of a hat, but with each update, there was little or no reaction. Because of the disease, her emotions had become quite suppressed, so it would take a lot to get her upset. Since she and her mother had been close, I would temper my medical updates so that I could keep her informed but not upset her. No matter what I said or how I said it, my news got little or no reaction.

I decided that maybe Lynne did not understand whom I was talking about. I had been using the three names interchangeably, as we all had for years. One day, I sat down before one of the medical updates and asked, "Do you know who Mary is?" She replied with a definite maybe in her voice, but she eventually did say yes. I asked the same question about the name "Grandma" and received the same response. I then asked about "Mom" and again got the same response. Then I asked if she knew that they were all the same person. From Lynne's initial response, it was obvious that she did not realize that these three names were attached to a single person. After I established that these three people were just a single person, I then only used "your mom" or "your mother" when referring to my mother-in-law and advised other family members to do the same.

Over the next few days, I did a Grandma, Mary, and Mom reinforcement drill a few times just to make sure that Lynne understood. Having felt I had cleared the confusion, I was confident that the next step, while it certainly had the potential to be difficult, could be accomplished without too much undue confusion. I had to tell Lynne that her mother was near death.

But in order to tell Lynne about her mother's situation (having seen the confusion of the names), I first had to establish whether Lynne knew what it meant when someone died or passed away. I posed the question and patiently waited for an answer. She thought for a few moments and responded in her typical halting, stuttering way, "They go away." I felt satisfied that she had at least some understanding, so I did not see any need to continue with a reinforcement drill like I had with the names.

My next step was to put "Mom" and "death" into a manageable format so that Lynne could understand. So with a well-crafted, well-rehearsed speech, I told Lynne that her mother was very, very sick, and the doctor said that she would probably pass away very soon. With what I hoped was not too much information for Lynne to digest, I could see the wheels turning. I was waiting for a reaction of some type. I sat with her for what seemed like hours but was in reality only a few moments of nervous anticipation.

With almost no warning, Lynne started wailing. Crying does not even come close to the level of grief she demonstrated. She cried so hard that she started hyperventilating. It was really the type of reaction I would have expected if Mary's situation had occurred before the Alzheimer's. The whole crying event lasted for about ten minutes. And when the crying was over, it was over. It was like she had just turned it off like a light switch. The pre-AD Lynne would have sat and whimpered for thirty minutes or more after a crying jag such as she had just experienced.

When Mary passed a few days later, I very gently told Lynne that, like we had talked about, her mother had died. While I was preparing for another tsunami, she looked at me and said flatly, "Oh?" And not a tear was shed—not then and not since. When I speak of her mother to other people while Lynne is present, I speak openly of her mother's death and still get little or no reaction from Lynne. I have even gone as far as to ask her or tell her about her mother's passing, and I still get little more than a blank stare.

While Lynne was still able to work safely in the kitchen, I found a recipe for an oriental fish dish that she was willing to try. So one day, I set out the recipe, ingredients, measuring spoons, and the pan to cook it in and left Lynne to measure, mix, and prepare the dish. I left the room so she would not feel pressured or turn to me to do the job for her. She eventually came to me and asked where the ground ginger was because it was not on the counter or in the cabinet with the other spices. In all the preparation, it had been moved behind something else. I recovered it and left her to finish the dish.

As the dish was cooking, I thought to myself, *The aroma is familiar but not what I expected.* But this was a new recipe, so I really didn't know what to expect. When dishing up the fish, I still didn't recognize the aroma, but it was still familiar. The first bite told me that Lynne had modified the recipe. Instead of the ground ginger that was called for in the recipe, she had used ground cloves. Not wanting to hurt her feelings because she had worked so hard, I ate the next bite and the next until I could no longer feel my tongue.

The only time I witnessed Lynne truly angry was when we went to the animal shelter, looking for a new puppy. We found an eight-week-old ball of fluff that Lynne instantly fell in love with. After completing the adoption paperwork, the shelter official interviewed us to determine our suitably for this or any dog. As the interview progressed, it became apparent that the adoption process would take a few days so a representative of the shelter could do a home visit before releasing the puppy. With each passing moment, Lynne was becoming less and less patient with the shelter official—to the point where she was quite vocal and irritated with the whole process. I kept trying to calm her while I explained the reason for the home visit. But my words were not heard because Lynne was too busy loudly defending us to all of the staff and visitors of the shelter.

After a few years in business, Lynne and I determined that we needed a larger, more professional office in a better location. We visited an office building a block from our little office and checked out three of the available suites that matched our size and use requirements. After a quick tour, we decided the offices on the south side of the building would be better for us. These offices had a better view with fewer tall buildings, good view of a portion of historic Fairfax, and an unobstructed view of the funeral home and small city cemetery. While in the third office, we discussed the pluses and minuses of the three offices while standing in the portion of the office overlooking the street. Lynne, without cracking a smile, said, "At least you'll have fresh flowers every day."

Lynne—Published Author!

This story appeared in *Legions of Light*, Issue 31, in 2001. This was Lynne's only published story, which was written before she presented her first very discrete Alzheimer's symptoms. I felt that a little fiction might be a good way to try to forget, if for just a moment, the surrounding nonfiction. So I hope you enjoy my wife's first (and, unfortunately, last) published writing effort.

Snow Bound

by

Lynne Tutor

Alone in the frilly bedroom, Amy pulled on the borrowed nightgown. The room smelled like freshly cut lilacs. "I can't believe Dad thinks it's snowing too much."

Amy's father had told her to spend the night at Brenda's. That meant Amy would be sleeping in a strange bed in a strange house. She didn't want to wear someone else's nightgown, especially Brenda's. Brenda James was the biggest girl she knew. Brenda was at least five foot eight and three hundred pounds.

Amy shoved the sleeves of her borrowed nightgown up to her wrists and looked in the mirror. "I've been swallowed by a giant, pink flannel tent. I hope it doesn't strangle me while I'm sleeping."

"Amy, are you all right?" Brenda asked.

Amy jumped and spun around as Brenda filled the now open doorway. "Yes," Amy said softly. Her cheeks suddenly felt hot; she wondered if Brenda had heard anything. "I'm just angry with Dad for not letting me come home. I've driven in snow storms before, and it's only ten miles."

Brenda frowned and said, "In case you didn't notice we were driving in a blizzard. We could barely see past the hood. If you didn't want to stay here and wait out the storm, why did you call home?"

"I just wanted them to know that I left the cast party early and I was on my way," Amy said, trying to sound convincing.

"Well, like it or not, you're stuck with me," Brenda giggled. "You look like a little girl playing dress-up," Brenda said as she turned off the lights and worked her way into the patchwork sleeping bag on the floor. "Good night, Amy. By the way, that was a terrific performance you gave tonight."

"Thanks." Amy lay in bed, replaying the evening's events. *Why did you ever offer anyone a ride?* she thought. *If it weren't for all those stops on the way through town, I'd be home now.*

Brenda was in some of Amy's classes this year as well as in the senior play with her. Even so, Amy really didn't know her. Amy looked at the shadowy mount on the floor and shuddered. *I've done my best to avoid speaking to her or her fat friends. And she gave up her bed for me,* Amy thought as she rolled over, pulled the covers up under her chin, and closed her eyes.

She heard a soft, unfamiliar voice in the distance, "Girls, it's time to get up." She burrowed deeper into the warm covers, squeezed her eyes closed even tighter, and hoped the voice would go away. "Girls, it's time to get up," Mrs. James said sweetly as she opened the bedroom door.

"Daddy will drive you to school if you help shovel the driveway."

Amy peeked out from beneath the covers, looked at the patchwork mountain, and remembered where she was.

Brenda smiled and said, "Good morning, Amy."

"Hi," Amy responded as she turned her attention to Mrs. James. "I can't go to school. I don't have anything to wear except my party dress."

Mrs. James smiled and said, "We can find you something, dear."

Amy looked at the rotund Mrs. James. "That's all right; I'll just wear my party dress."

A few minutes later, Brenda placed a pair of faded jeans, a bright red sweater, and a braided cloth belt on the bed. "I found some clothes for you to wear. They're the smallest I have."

Amy felt awkward when she realized Brenda wasn't apologizing for her size, just stating a fact. "Thanks," Amy said without looking at Brenda.

"I'll be outside, helping my Dad shovel the driveway," Brenda said as she turned to leave the room.

She acts like being fat is normal. How can she look like that and still be so confident? Amy wondered.

A heavy silence filled the small, sunlit room. Crawling out of bed, she looked at Brenda's clothes and almost cried. *Stop feeling sorry for yourself. You're stuck here for now, so make the best of it. After all, it's better to wear big jeans that a party dress when shoveling snow.*

She dressed quickly; ran a brush through her tangled, chestnut hair; tightened the belt to keep the jeans from falling off; and headed for the stairs.

Amy opened the door and squinted at the blinding sunlight bouncing off the sea of snow. *It's so much brighter than last night's stage lights,* she thought; then she saw the wall of snow surrounding her car.

"The plows have been busy already!" she yelled toward Brenda and her father. "It's going to be tough digging my car out."

"If you wait until after school, I'll help you," Brenda shouted.

Amy looked at Brenda, thought about spending another night with her, and frowned. "I'm not going to school. I'm going home."

"Amy, be reasonable. We got at least eighteen inches of snow last might," Brenda said as she walked toward Amy. "I'm going to school even if you don't, and I don't think you can dig your car out alone. Thanks to the snow plows, there's heavy, hard-packed snow piled up so high you probably won't get the car door open. Your car isn't going anywhere today."

Amy knew Brenda was right, but she didn't want to admit it. "I can't go to school in my party dress."

"Yes, you can. Just wear your dress to school, and act as if it's perfectly normal. Besides, the girls in their jeans and sweaters will be jealous when you come to school all dressed up. All it takes is confidence. Everyone respects confidence and the strength to be different. You don't have to be confident; just act as if you are. You're a good actress; you can do it," Brenda said with authority and returned to her shoveling. "Besides, I'll bet we get all the help we need to shovel your car out once the boys find out you're stranded."

"Okay. You win. I'll go to school." *I think I like this girl,* Amy thought as she smiled, picked up a spare shovel, and headed for the driveway.

Hazel's Background

My mother was born and raised in Harnett County, North Carolina. She was the oldest of three girls born to my grandparents, Marvin and Lena Mangum. Raised in a farm family in Depression-era North Carolina, my mother developed a strong sense of family, understood the necessity of hard work, and appreciated the value of a dollar.

After attending Louisburg College and completing a course of study at a business school in Raleigh, my mother began her civilian Army career at Fort Bragg. In 1941, she moved to Washington, DC, and after a short stint in the private sector, joined the ranks of the federal government. After a short stay in the temporary government buildings (that stood for over fifty years) in Washington, my mother was part of one of the first groups to move into the new and still-under-construction headquarters of the Department of Defense—the Pentagon. She certainly found her niche as she worked for the Army between federal service and as a consultant for over fifty-five years. She was recognized as the subject matter expert on one of the computer systems supporting the Joint Chiefs of Staff.

On the family side of her life, after the death of her sister, "Buddy," in 1992, Mom decided to reunite her third sister, Frances Louise, with my grandparents. Frances Louise was five months old when she died in 1924. "The Baby" was buried at Piney Grove Baptist Church Cemetery. So in 1995, my mother put the wheels in motion to have the baby's remains moved to my grandparents' resting place so they would finally be together. Because of my mother's inability to travel and the diagnosis of Alzheimer's, she was never able to visit the baby's new resting site. The level of pride she experienced in this labor of love was seldom spoken of, but you could see it in my mother's eyes. She had done something that some thought was stupid or wasteful for her long-deceased sister and their parents that had no monetary measure—just an overwhelming sense of joy.

I was twelve years old when my father was diagnosed with cancer and thirteen when he died. I knew he was sick. I knew he wasn't doing well. I found out that he was dying a few hours after he died. At about three o'clock in the morning, my mother had to wake me from a sound sleep to give me the news that my father had passed away. She had waited six months to tell me that he was going to die. It escapes me to this day why she could not wait a few more hours to tell me instead of waking me in the middle the night. I think the news, as bad as it was, could have waited, since it had waited for so long before. And I remember that morning as clearly as if it happened this morning. I also remember watching her watch him fade away—how she steadfastly stayed by my father's bedside throughout the six months he lay dying at Fairfax Hospital.

After the doctor determined that my father had a malignant brain tumor and that even with surgery and radiation, he would not survive, my mother ordered the doctor not to tell him. And she had no intention of telling him either. Nor did she tell me that he was dying for fear I would let it slip, since I visited him nearly every day he was in the hospital. She told me several years later that she never told him of his fate, but she was sure he knew based on something a family friend said after visiting my father at the hospital.

I did not realize it at the time, but I had a front-row seat to what to do and not do when observing my mother throughout my father's decline and death. This is part of what defines my desire to care for my best friend and the love of my life. It is my mission as long as we draw breath. As I have often been heard to say, I am absolute in my resolve. I will care for Lynne, no matter what sacrifices I must make, for as long as it takes.

———

After my grandmother had passed in 1984, my mother dutifully packed up the remainder of my grandmother's belongings, including all the textiles and kitchenware. When she arrived home, the textiles were carefully stowed in closets and dressers. Every spring, all the sheets would come out to be washed, ironed, folded, and returned to their assigned closet or dresser. This ritual continued every year without fail until 2005—the spring that mom broke her hip.

One fall, there was an unusually early frost predicted. Lynne and I had a very productive garden, as usual, and this early frost was going to ruin the last of the crops. We did not have enough of our own sheets to cover everything, so I foolishly asked my mother if I could borrow some of her sheets. You would have thought I had asked for a kidney! Actually, a kidney would have been easier. To say I received a resounding no would truly be an understatement. She prized these sheets like they were the crown jewels. Of all the sheets—an untold, unimaginable quantity—not one sheet fit any of the beds in her home or any in mine. During the 2007 cleanout, all the sheets were piled in the middle the living room floor. There were four piles of plain white cotton sheets; each pile was more than three feet deep.

The kitchenware that she brought from my grandmother's found its way into a storage cabinet that my mother specifically bought to entomb these pieces of cookware. My grandparents had owned and operated a mom-and-pop restaurant for decades. These pieces were institutional cookware, not decorative, and certainly not the size a single person cooking for one would ever use. From 1984 until 2007, these pieces sat in this storage cabinet, untouched until the big cleanout.

So what happened to the sheets and kitchenware? With the exception of a few pieces of the kitchenware that I kept and use, it was all boxed up by the girls who helped with the cleanout and shipped back to their families in their native El Salvador. (At least that's the story I was told, and it's none of my business anyway.) So after twenty-three years of safekeeping, the sheets that my mother prized so highly and the kitchenware that had gone into hiding for nearly a quarter of a century finally found a home and are probably being used by somebody.

———✵◦◦◦✵◦✵◦◦◦✵———

My father died in 1965, and as a veteran, he was buried at Arlington National Cemetery (ANC). His funeral was well attended by family, friends, and coworkers. The service was held at a funeral home just a few blocks from our home, followed by the police-led processional the sixteen-miles to the cemetery. A brief graveside service complete with mourners, the honor guard, a few nosy tourists, and the folded American flag closed the funeral for my dad.

When my mother had her arrangements made, she envisioned a simple but elegant service at the same funeral home, complete with a close family friend delivering the heartfelt eulogy, the minister from my grandmother's church, a cousin playing the organ, and scores of mourners in attendance. Following the service, the carefully selected pallbearers would move her remains to the waiting hearse. The wailing sirens of the police motorcycles leading the procession would herald her approach to her final resting place with my father.

A few flaws came to light when the end came. My mother, while an important figure during her many years at the Pentagon, was still just a civilian and the dependent of an average World War II Marine Corps Private First Class. To put it simply, as a veteran's dependent, you are pretty much the lowest rung on the ladder at ANC. The deceased and the family are still treated with great respect at ANC, but veteran's dependents are their lowest priority, especially with the number of funerals they have on any given day, as the veteran population ages and we continue to have soldiers dying in the field of battle. Therefore, you wait in line—not literally, but wait you must. My mother died on

May 5 but was not buried until June 29. So much for the screaming motorcycles from Fairfax to Arlington.

The funeral she was hoping for—simple but elegant, with the ensuing police-escorted processional to ANC—was reduced to a viewing and a brief graveside service conducted by, of all things, after fifty-five years of Army service, a navy chaplain. Both events were sparsely attended, as I had expected. The viewing garnered only eight people, including Lynne and Nichole, who were there for just a few minutes. The graveside service, on the other hand, brought together a total of thirteen people. Even though the number was small, it did represent nearly every aspect of my mother's eighty-nine years on this earth. After all, it's the quality of the people, not the quantity, which counts for so much at this moment in time.

The reasons for the low turnout, which I had expected, were quite simple and were the driving force behind reducing her funeral plans the way I did. Most of the relatives she grew up with were either dead or unable to travel the three hundred miles from North Carolina to Northern Virginia. Even though she worked with thousands of uniformed and civilian Army and Defense Department employees, she had lost touch with most of them—and again, many of them were unable to travel or had passed away. The people she still had contact with were scattered across the country, and much of her contact with them over the years had been little more than a Christmas card, an e-mail note, or a rare telephone call.

I feel confident that the low turnout by her friends in the area was simply due to the fact that she had called many of them so frequently I am sure they grew tired of the same AD-generated questions and stories. I was sure that the turnout was going to be low since very few of her friends attempted to contact her after she moved to Happy Valley. In the months following her relocation, there were no messages on her answering machine from friends or family, no calls to me wondering why she wasn't answering her telephone, no e-mails to her account or mine regarding her absence, and no cards or letters except from the charities she once donated to. She had disappeared from their lives, and apparently none of her friends seemed to notice or really care.

———— ᴡᴡ∘ᴏᴇᴦᴏ᷍ᴏᴦᴇᴏᴏᴡᴡ ————

Happy Valley would occasionally have drives around the neighborhood so the residents would have a change of scenery. I never could understand taking a group of dementia patients out of the building on such a drive when they only would have one or two staff members accompanying a dozen regular residents and dementia patients.

One of these drive events occurred late in the afternoon, which for my mother, was the most cognitively challenging part of her day. I arrived just as they were leaving, and from my previous experience with these outings, they would usually be gone about forty-five minutes, so I decided to wait in my mother's room. When the customary return time had more than doubled, I became concerned that maybe something had happened to the small bus the facility used, so I went to find out if anything had happened—whether they had been involved in an accident, the bus had broken down, or they were stuck in the legendary Washington rush hour traffic.

I was hard-pressed to find any of the staff. I eventually was told by one of the aides that everybody was at the front door, trying to get one of the dementia patients back into the building. My imagination did not need to run wild. I was confident that the dementia patient in question and I shared the same last name. As I reached the front lobby, they had finally convinced her to come into the facility after coaxing, encouraging, and negotiating with her for over thirty minutes to come in and wait for someone to come pick her up. Her reason for not wanting to come in the building was simple: "I don't live here, and I want to go home." It was many months before they would allow her access to the other portions of the facility—even with an escort—and they certainly did not allow her to go on one of these neighborhood tours.

Hazel's Alzheimer's

T he situation we often find ourselves in is understanding the dementia victim's thoughts and actions. My mother lived in the same room at Happy Valley for nearly two and a half years, and with the exception of two brief escapes, a few trips to the doctor, visits to the emergency room connected to the facility, and a few drives around the neighborhood, she never left Happy Valley. But in her mind, she had been there for three days—not two or four, always three days. She had seen and noted the change of seasons, but with the short-term memory loss, she did not remember anything more than the dead tree in the landscape. Forever the pessimist, she always said, "Someone needs to cut that dead tree down before it falls and hurts someone."

While at Happy Valley, my mother was often agitated to a point just short of combativeness. This near-combativeness included using her cane to "get the attention of the staff" by tapping on the glass surrounding the nurse's station, resulting in hundreds of pieces of nurse's station glass flying in all directions. The answer was, of course, to take her cane and drug her up to the point where she could still function and would not be a problem to the staff or the other residents. This was done under the guidance of the geriatric psychiatrist who stopped by for a visit on occasion. I understand the reasons, and while I am not a fan of the concept, the small staff had fifteen to eighteen dementia patients to care for and keep under control. The drug route was the best way to handle the situation. The drugs mellowed out my mother, which helped break down her agitation and resistance to the staff, to a certain degree, which allowed them to better assist her and make her stay at least a little more tolerable.

Nearly every day for the first year my mother lived at Happy Valley, she would pack all of her belongings, since she was ready to go home. No matter how many times I put everything away and explained that she would have to stay longer, I would return the next day to find two neatly packed boxes containing some of her Happy Valley clothes and personal items. Even when I snuck the empty boxes out and instructed the staff to not let her have any more, she would still find replacements.

When she could no longer find boxes, she would neatly fold everything and stack it all on the dresser. Then while she waited for me or someone to come in the afternoon, she would wander like a lost puppy, carrying a few items—usually the photographs and her slippers. Eventually, she did stop packing, but she would still occasionally gather a few items and then pace back and forth all afternoon, impatiently waiting for her ride home.

While my mother lived at Happy Valley, the facility was apparently on wheels. On numerous occasions, she would tell me that this was her house in any one of three locations in Virginia, her parents' house in two locations in North Carolina, the apartment she shared with an aunt in 1941 in Washington, and several times, the basement of the Pentagon, where she had worked for several decades. She also apparently was living at the firehouse, but I never could determine the location of the firehouse or understand why she picked the firehouse, as she never lived in or near any firehouse. She was also often convinced that she was in the hospital, awaiting surgery. But no matter where she was or when it was, there was one thing that was an absolute, carved-in-stone fact—she needed to leave, and she was not going to stay any longer than she had to.

Before my mother moved to Happy Valley, she began receiving telephone calls from my grandmother—"Mama called, and she needs help"—and then the short-distance wandering began. I am no expert in the field of wandering, even if such an expert exists, but I am sure my mother's wandering after she started receiving these imagined telephone calls from her mother was actually her looking for my grandparents' house or the restaurant my grandparents owned years ago. I am also not an expert in the field of telecommunications, but I am sure my grandmother was not calling, since she died some twenty years earlier. Strangely enough, my mother never received any of these "I need help" telephone calls from any other person, living or dead.

Since she had never been one to walk very much, coupled with the recent broken hip, my mother's wandering never got her too far. Her wandering usually landed her at my front door or at one of the neighbors' homes. All things being equal, at least I wasn't chasing her all over town, calling the police, or finding her dead in the woods. Her little journeys would occur any time of the day but usually in the late afternoon or early evening, which I believe was part of her sundowning. (More information on sundowning later.) My biggest concern was the large quantity of cut-through traffic in our neighborhood—and she lived on the corner of the two busiest streets. Another concern I had with her wandering was that no matter what the temperature, she never wore anything more than a short-sleeve cotton shirt, lightweight cotton slacks, and a pair of slippers that she swore belonged to my grandfather, who died in 1968. No matter how cold—even with ice and snow on the ground—she would be out, walking or wandering, wearing just enough to not get arrested.

I had been warned that eventually, I would become just a nameless face—another forgotten person from my mother's disappearing past. Before I moved her to Happy Valley, she had started having episodes of not knowing me. After she moved, of course, the frequency increased to almost daily, which also came as no surprise. But no matter who I was, I became her lifeline to the past—not just retelling stories and events from our past, but usually becoming whomever she wanted to talk to at that particular moment in time.

Every afternoon, I would go to Happy Valley to sit and visit with my mother. Understand that, even though I had not changed my appearance in decades and would be sitting in front of her with just the two of us in her room, she often had no idea I was her son, a relative, or even a neighbor. Many times, she told the staff—sometimes just moments following my daily visit—the reason I never came to see her was because I must be in jail again. One day, she even told me that her son was in jail when she thought I was someone else. Point of information: the closest I have ever been in jail was to bail out my stepchildren—Nichole for a traffic ticket and Mason for a variety of things.

I became an ever-expanding list of people from my mother's past. On any given day, I could be her father, her husband (talk about a sticky situation), the brother she never had, her brother-in-law's brother (but never her brother-in-law), cousins, friends, and former coworkers. All of these people had their stories to tell, many of which she told as I led her in the conversation so I could understand whom she was talking about and how they fit in her life. Every person I became apologized for not having come to see her and missed seeing her over the appropriate period of time. I never corrected her, never told her she was wrong, and played the parts as well as I could to keep from upsetting her. I played my parts well except for one time. I could not play the part of her sister, Buddy, with a straight face; nor did I tell her that her sister had passed away several years earlier.

I became quite the storyteller, assuming the identity of people whom, in some cases, I never knew—either because they had died long before I would have met them or because they were people she had worked with whom I never met. The key to my success in this "entertainment" of my memory-stricken mother was to listen to not only what she said, but also how she said it. I would gauge her attitude toward the person I was playing to determine whether I should be a relative, close friend, or casual acquaintance.

On the few days that my mother recognized me after her entry into Happy Valley, questions would often come along as to what I did for a living. She never had been comfortable with my stay-at-home, self-employed lifestyle, so to keep her from being upset about my employment situation (because taking care of Lynne 24/7 was not a real job), I made up jobs for myself—and sometimes for the people that I had become—to satisfy her delusions and confusions and to fill dead air in our conversations. Sometimes I was a character from a television show or movie, a person in the news, or a combination of both. A few times, I became who she was when she worked at the Pentagon, and she was none the wiser. No character, real or imagined, was ever a superhero, a rock star, a Pulitzer Prize winner, or anything else too hard to believe.

As I developed these characters and played the parts of people whose names I never knew before, I would keep mental notes on who they were to her so that if I became that person again, I would know how to play the part more convincingly with less input from her. This is where the concept of revisionist history or creative storytelling can be an effective tool in the caregiver's toolbox. Remember, your audience has difficultly remembering what happened in the past—especially the recent past—so any mistakes you make will most likely not be discovered by your loved one. If they catch you in a mistake, keep it in mind for the next time you need to tell the story, because the subject will likely come around again and again. And remember, if they catch you in a mistake, they are always right—no matter what.

It's up to you how great you make yourself or how much you revise the past, so you always have a happy ending. And that's one thing I always had—no matter how bad the ending was in real life, there was always a happy ending. Isn't that the way it's supposed to be—whether you are living in the real world or the deluded fantasy world of a dementia patient?

Like I said earlier, I am a storyteller. For my mother, I had become the Scheherazade of Happy Valley just to keep her content during the closing chapters of her life in a home that she was always a stranger in. But a funny thing happened along the way while playing the various people from her past. I actually learned something about her past, and sometimes I was a bit surprised by some of the people and events in her life. Occasionally, though, unbeknownst to her, Lynne and I got a few laughs at her expense over some of my recreations or resurrections of people whom neither of us ever knew and likely never would.

Nearly every day after she went to Happy Valley, my mother asked about friends and relatives from her North Carolina past, most of whom had long ago died or had forgotten about her. It got so wearisome that I started telling her that I had talked with them recently. They were always just fine, going on vacation or something from real life that would sell it. Sometimes I would even tell her a story to give her the impression that I was truly keeping up with the family and friends who were not keeping up with her. The moral to the story is simple but at the same time complex—you do what you have got to do to help your loved one through the end of his or her life because it's the right thing to do. But be careful not to develop a Jesus complex because you keep bringing dead people back to life.

Mary/Grandma/Mom

In all this talk of my caregiving duties for my wife and my mother, I have not touched on my first caregiving job. Lynne's mother, Mary, lived with us for over twenty years until she remarried at the age of ninety-three—yes, ninety-three! She met and married Cliff, a young buck of eighty-eight who lived eleven houses up the street and had since 1961.

Jenny, our letter carrier, told Mary about Cliff in late June. His wife had passed away, and Jenny thought that since the two of them were alone, maybe they could chat on the telephone or have lunch together occasionally. Mary was reluctant at first but agreed to at least talk with Cliff. They were married in October of the same year. They had a few good years together but passed a few months apart in 2010. Their time together is another excellent example of how God sometimes works in mysterious ways. Had Mary still been living with us, I would have had three desperately ill people to juggle. And as high-maintenance as my mother was and Lynne can be, Mary often beat them both by a mile.

While Mary had been diagnosed with Parkinson's disease very early, the majority of her medical problems did not involve the Parkinson's. Mary was the poster child for eye problems. That made me her medical transport in the beginning. But I rapidly became the medical liaison when she could no longer understand (if she ever did) what the ophthalmologists were telling her about her eye problems and what could be done to improve the situation. Her many appointments had me driving her, sitting with her in the waiting room, accompanying her into the exam rooms, talking with the doctors, and then translating what the doctors said once we got home. For a time, I spoke fairly fluent layman's ophthalmology. That was before I switched my specialty to neurology.

People

Our cast of characters, in no particular order, includes the same type of people and personalities you likely have in your own family and circle of friends. Like everybody else, we have the ones who enjoy their work and the ones for whom work is just a means to an end, ones who enjoy their play and ones who enjoy play too much, ones who put family first and ones who feel family should be avoided except when financial support is needed, ones who consider all options when making decisions and ones who dive in head-first without checking the depth of the water, ones who keep their eye on the ball and ones who can't even find the ballpark—a typical collection of folks, probably no different from yours. And if you are in my family or circle of friends, I hope you know who you are. If you don't know who you are in this list, give me a call or send me an e-mail.

Let's start the character rollout with me. Since this is really about me and how I have cared for my wife, mother, and mother-in-law over the years, I won't dwell on myself at this point. I will say that you may note throughout my book some sarcasm, strong opinions, and deep hatred. And while diplomacy is not one of my strengths, I can be diplomatic enough to temper whatever comes out of my mouth—but only if absolutely necessary. Try to remember that I am very much a black-and-white sort of person, especially when it comes to people—not too much gray area or tolerance for stupidity here. But know this—when it comes to my devotion to Lynne, I am in this battle to the end, and I take no prisoners.

Nichole, Lynne's firstborn, is a truly wonderful person whose biggest fault can be summed up in one word—*later.* "Don't put off until tomorrow what you can avoid until next week" was Nichole's way of life until she found out that being a wife, mother, and stepmother usually does not allow for a lot of procrastination. She is certainly not an angel in the helping-Dad-take-care-of-Mom scenario, but she tries to help whenever possible. But with a house full of people to care for and clean up after, her logistics issues are never-ending. When she has the time—and she has so little time to spare—she is a truly generous and caring person. She is smart as a whip, sometimes a bit naïve, but always eager to help when she can.

As much as it pains us all to say, Nichole had a practice run at marriage. To make this is brief as possible, as the marriage was brief, to say the least, she and her longtime boyfriend married and shared the same address for a short while. One day, she came home to empty closets, a pile of bills he had run up using her formerly good credit, and a note.

During and after the divorce, Nichole and her three dogs lived on a horse farm in Hume, Virginia, in a house that we lovingly called the little hovel on the prairie. The place was built in the 1850s and was originally used as slave quarters. For its age, the humble cottage was in fairly good condition although it was conveniently located close to the edge of the earth, so getting there featured a bumpy drive down a pothole-filled dirt road and fording a stream on the property. But the view more than made up for the inconvenience and lack of amenities. This little place offered Nichole the quiet and solitude—not to mention the view—that she needed to recover from a less-than-happy marriage.

She lived in the hovel for a few years, getting her life back on track emotionally and financially. She didn't date much while living on the farm. Inviting someone back to her place was not really practical, since this lovely little home was several miles off the beaten track—not the type of ice breaker most folks are looking for in a new relationship. But when Nichole was ready, she and her two dogs moved to an apartment (on a paved road), and she started dating more seriously. This is where a new character entered our lives. Nichole met James at a Christian singles' mixer, and the story is quite varied as to how long James was in the picture before we actually had a chance to meet. The reason for her delay in our meeting was that she didn't want to jinx it.

James can often be described in a single word—*focused*. Organized to a point just short of obsession he and Nichole are a well-matched team. Although they married in 2007, in some ways, they are still in the newlywed phase, even though there are teenagers and an infant running about. They met, married, and had a child while James was still in the US Navy. Shortly after they married, he was transferred to Norfolk, Virginia, and eventually, because of this terrorism thing we have all heard about, he was out of the country on temporary duty for eighteen months. After twenty years of service in the Navy, he retired, moved the family to the Washington area, and with a solid, in-demand background, found a good job quite easily.

And in the finest tradition set forth by her mother and her grandmother, Nichole married a younger man. James, like both of Mary's husbands and me, the husband is younger than the wife.

Could I have saved the best for last? You be the judge. Mason, Lynne's youngest, continues to baffle us all. Of the many not-so-kind words that would best describe Mason, *estranged* is probably the least offensive. His desire to be a loving, caring family member seems to always take a backseat to his work and play—but mostly his play. He currently works as a server at a national chain casual-dining establishment—just another in a very long succession of restaurants he has worked at as a waiter, assistant manager, or manager over the past twenty years. But when away from the restaurant, he spends most of his time playing fantasy games. He rarely visits any of the family, even though Lynne and I live less than fifteen minutes away and Nichole about forty-five minutes away. He has always just lost or just broken his most recent cell phone about the same time you just left three messages about something important. He is always too sick or too busy so he does not have to interact with the family.

Some say he is trying to distance himself from his dying mother and avoiding what the disease has done to her, choosing to remember her the way she was. This is an interesting theory we all would be happy to embrace, but he has been this way (and worse) since age fifteen. But as bad as he is and has been, Nichole, James, and I continue to reach out to him, letting him know we still care and that we are willing to help him get his life on track without judging him for his past indiscretions.

While Lynne was still able to understand things like time, it bothered her that Mason was seldom around and that he did not seem to care what was happening to her or any other family members. Eventually, whenever she spoke about the kids, it was always Nichole and "No Name." As the disease progressed, and the people in Lynne's memory started to fade, Mason was the first family member to become consistently forgotten. She still does occasionally remember him, but the love that she once had for him has certainly faded. While she does not remember Mason's many teenage antics (another kind word), she does remember that he was not an angel, that he made several questionable choices in life, and that we were often suspicious of him and the life he was living. When she does remember him, she still wonders what happened to drive him away. For some time, she thought it was our fault that he turned out the way he has. Here is where memory loss can be a benefit. Fortunately, the disease has erased the guilt that Lynne felt about how Mason turned out.

At one point, I offered a monetary inducement to encourage his participation in our little family. (That sounds like a bribe to me too!) All he had to do was visit us for one hour every month, and the same with Nichole and her family. There were no conditions other than his physical presence with his family members. All I was asking for was a total of two hours out of his life every month, not including drive time. I told him when we made the agreement that the only excuse I would accept for his not coming to visit us or his sister was his death. I also told him that should he miss a visit with either of us, my offer to increase his net worth would be voided.

James and Nichole felt that I had set myself up for a large monetary loss. I knew it was the safest bet I could ever make based on Mason's track record and his desire to not always do what's best for himself. In his typical commitment to excellence, especially in family matters, he managed to meet these very simple conditions for two months. My offer was made in March. At the end of April and May, he managed to visit. But June came and went with no visit. From March through December, Mason visited us a total of six times—enough said.

Our family has been quite blessed with wonderful pets throughout the years. Through our time together, our four-legged children have included cats—Angel, Smokey, Keishu, Cricket, and Dusty. The list of dogs is shorter—Goggles, Ginger, and Genie—because we felt one dog was good for bonding with the family without jealousy factors between multiple dogs. We also found room in our hearts for two house rabbits, Harvey and Smudgy. Genie and Dusty are still with us, and of all our pets, they are perfect for the situation we find ourselves in now.

Dusty is a fifteen-pound, buff-colored Tom that, like most of our pets, was adopted from a rescue organization. He is getting up in years and spends most this time doing what cats do best—eating, sleeping, and pooping. He is quite low-key and seldom bothers Lynne but is quite eager to be petted when Lynne can see him, touch him, and not step on him.

Genie is a dream dog. She is an all-black, sixty-pound Chow, Lab, and Border Collie mix that also came from a rescue organization. She keeps the barking to a minimum, does not get on the furniture as a rule, and knows that when Lynne is up and moving, it's best to move to a safe place.

When I leave the house, Genie moves into position so that she can protect Lynne. She stations herself within a few feet of Lynne for as long as I am out of the house. That is all her; that's not a command I taught her. She just feels the need to help out by staying close to Lynne. She could teach some humans a thing or two about caring.

One morning, I had to deal with a tow truck driver who was picking up Nichole and James's car from our driveway. While I was outside, Lynne was sitting on the love seat, listening to the television. I was outside for about fifteen minutes. When I returned, there sat Lynne on the love seat, as I had left her. Snuggled up next to her on Lynne's little love seat lay Genie in protect mode. She certainly was not comfortable because of the tight fit, but she was doing what came naturally to her—protecting Lynne, since I was not in the house.

There is a very large and quite diverse population of caregivers in the caregiving business, no matter what the illness or condition, but it really only comes down to four types—the ones who can't do enough to help their loved one; the ones who can't run away fast enough or far enough but always claim to be there to help; those who care enough to criticize everything that you are doing, but are never there to help; and the ones who say, "Have somebody else handle it." Except for the first type, they all have the same caregiving concept in common—put the victim in a home or push the victim off onto another relative; just get someone else to take care of them.

The first caregiver group is hard to find unless you venture into their world because they are usually too busy to come to you. They can be found in the trenches, doing their best, trying to keep their loved one clean, safe, fed, and comfortable with little regard for themselves. And if you are a caregiver giving care, the hours are usually longer because you not only have to care for the patient, but also handle other duties, like housekeeping, laundry, and all those other pesky responsibilities that seem to occur in real life. And some caregivers have more people than just their patient to care for. They can also have grandparents, parents, spouses, and children who need help in the real world.

Now let's talk about you, your circle of contacts, your AD victim, and the possibility of embarrassment—especially out in the real world. First and foremost, if you get embarrassed about the disease, any uncontrollable outburst because of it, or just can't deal with any element of the disease, *get over it!* Or find someone who can deal with it. This disease is no different from any other disease. Your victim did not choose it from a "let's see what I can die from" list just to inconvenience or embarrass you. So if you or your family and friends can't deal with this disease, find a way sooner rather than later. Don't waste your time and the time that your victim has left trying to muster the courage to face the disease and its ramifications—and, of course, the inevitable.

Sometimes you may find it necessary to prepare your family, friends, and visitors for what to expect if they have not seen the toll a disease has taken on the victim since last they visited. I know from personal experience that Lynne aged five years by the calendar but looks as if she aged twenty-five years because of the stress of the disease. Try to get the visitors to avoid leading every story with, "Remember when . . ." Also be prepared for people to talk louder, since sick people are always assumed to be hard of hearing. Also be prepared to never see or hear from your visitors again. People are funny that way.

It is strange—even though I am essentially trapped in this house and rarely venture out except for a quick errand, I still meet people. Lynne and I, while we live very much like hermits, hidden away in our little Alzheimer's house, have managed to make a few new friends. Some are just voices on the telephone, some come to our door, and a few I have met in stores or offices. People I probably would not have met or spent time with otherwise, since until Lynne got sick, I usually would not strike up conversations with strangers. It is one of the personality traits I took over from Lynne when she was no longer able to chit-chat. Among the many, two very special people stand out.

In my non-travels, I have met a truly wonderful young man named Marc. He comes to our home monthly, bringing our supply of bottled water. He not only brings our water, but also kind words and truly the strongest prayer I have ever heard from a layperson. His prayers are truly from the heart and uplift the very tired spirit. His presence, even though it is brief, tells me that he was put on this route to show me that someone is watching out for us. I am truly proud to welcome him to my home and call him a friend.

We welcomed to our home two Mormon missionaries one afternoon. We agreed when they asked for a return visit. On their many subsequent visits each week, the missionaries would bring a member of the congregation. Often the congregant would have Alzheimer's experience, having lost a loved one to the disease. This is when our friend Amy entered our lives. She would frequently be the third member of the group. In our visits, we discovered that her late father was also an Alzheimer's victim. Our friendship grew quickly, and after the missionary visits ended, Amy would still find time in her very hectic schedule to stop in for a visit—not to encourage us to attend their church on Sunday, but as a good friend who just wants to talk, offer moral support, and occasionally mint chocolate chip ice cream, which is Lynne's favorite.

I have been told by many people that I go the extra mile and then some to care for my wife, and while my mother was still living at home, to care for her as best I could, all things considered. To that end, many people have indicated that I have set the bar for caregiving very high. I hope to tell the world, one person at a time, that should they be faced with this type of situation, they should wish to attain the level of dedication and commitment that I have with my loved ones once a terminal disease entered the picture.

Both my mother and Lynne, very special people in my life and the lives of others, suffered the cruelest of blows when Alzheimer's disease took over their lives. I hoped that their large number of friends and former coworkers would have taken at least a moment here and there to send an e-mail, a card, or a letter; make a telephone call; or God forbid, stop by for a quick visit.

These women made many friends the workplace. Some of these friendships withstood the test of time—some as much as forty years.

To some, my wife and my mother were more like surrogate mothers or sisters. I know that after leaving jobs, office friendships fade, but for the relationships that endure, you would think a simple "thinking of you" card, note, or e-mail would not be so tough. The people whom I direct this to should know who they are, and even though most are supposedly good Christians, they have either not attempted to contact us or have dropped by the wayside after an e-mail or two. For the few who did keep in touch, when my mother and Lynne were no longer able to respond, I took up the mantle to maintain contact.

I know I am from a time where attitudes toward others were quite different. I was taught that an offer of support, without strings attached, was what a friend gave to a friend or a neighbor gave to a neighbor—not out of some obligation but out of friendship.

For those who called my mother, my wife, and me friends, have a good, long look in the mirror. One day, you could be asking the same questions of your caregiver. If you are asking those questions, I hope you are crying the same tears my mother and my wife cried because you walked, ran, or just simply turned your back on a friend instead of taking a moment out of your busy life to offer a bit of emotional support. So little effort would have been needed to make these wonderful people feel just a bit better if but for just that moment in time. And trust me when I say this—I was not going to call on any of our supposed friends or errant family members for any physical, emotional, or financial assistance at any point in this ordeal.

Even though my first inclination is to tell these friends and family members to . . . but what good would it do? I do wish for them whatever they deserve, knowing full well that they feel they deserve more. The one thing I learned while watching these two very special people is that God is watching and will reward you for ignoring or willfully hurting others. And remember, you may get what you justly deserve when you least expect it.

Figure out how to explain to your mother, wife, or whomever you are taking care of why the people who used to be so close to them suddenly can't take time for them. Find out how to explain to them that the disease that is destroying them and stealing their very identity has sent their friends into hiding—probably because they lacked the backbone to come face-to-face with Alzheimer's, the death of a friend, or their own mortality. Find out how to tell them that the people who used to love them for who they were are now afraid of who they have become. I usually have an answer for most everything, but this one escapes me. So if you ever figure it out, let me know. I am always willing to learn.

I have indicated my lack of contentment with our former friends and long-absent relatives. I also have a level of dissatisfaction with the people whom we share this little slice of heaven we call Fairfax with—our neighbors. While each of them are decent and friendly people, they have not seen fit to offer any assistance at any point in our ordeal. I understand they have their lives, and I know they are busy with work, family, and the various activities that occur in suburbia. But that does not excuse (at least in my mind) not offering assistance with something as simple as offering to pick up something at the store.

The neighborhood we share is not the type that has a frequent turnover in owners. On our stretch of the street, I have been here the longest of any of the neighbors. I have lived on this block, between my current home and my parent's home, since September 1958. The people whom we call neighbors—or more accurately, the people we live near—have lived on this block for an average of about twelve years. I rarely see any of my neighbors, but when I do, I at least wave, and if possible, spend a few minutes chatting with them about various subjects no different than any other neighbors. And some may even ask how Lynne is doing and how I am doing while taking care of her.

We even have a neighbor who, no matter how bad you have it, has it worse, or one of her family members has it worse. (You probably have a neighbor like this also.) Even though she is an educated person and knows Lynne's diagnosis and prognosis, she always asks if Lynne is getting better. I applaud her for asking, but by now, I would think she would stop asking if Lynne is improving after I have told her many times that Lynne's time on this earth is coming to an early end.

While my mother was still living at home, I would walk back and forth from my house to hers every day, multiple times every day, at all hours of the day and night. The neighbors, in passing, might ask how one or both of my AD victims were doing but would never go out of their way to stop by or offer assistance. This is particularly disturbing since some of my neighbors have lived with family members who had Alzheimer's disease. They should understand that I could use at least a little emotional support, if nothing else.

A neighbor couple decided that they would bring both sets of parents to live with them and their four children. The wife, "Nancy," stopped in to visit us and also visited with my mother on occasion. Every morning, when Lynne took her customary walk, she would stop by this neighbor's house, chat with Nancy and the children if they were outside, and of course, visit with their mixed-breed dog. Lynne was one of the few people in the neighborhood who could safely approach this dog and did so nearly every morning.

Before Lynne and I started our first clinical trial, we asked Nancy if she would be an emergency contact for my mother while we were at Georgetown during the trial. She was agreeable to this, and nothing happened that required my mother to contact Nancy.

One afternoon, Nancy and her father were walking down the street, and I was taking my mother out a quick walk when we met at Mom's mailbox. Nancy announced that they had decided that they were going to bulldoze their existing house and rebuild. They estimated that the project would take approximately one year. I asked her to keep in touch with us, and if possible, bring the dog by for a visit so that Lynne and the dog might remain friends and we could maintain contact with the family.

We watched the demolition and reconstruction and were looking forward to the family's return once the house was complete. Once the family returned, several months passed, and Nancy made no attempt to reestablish contact. Even though she drove past our house frequently, she made no attempt to contact us. To my knowledge, Lynne and I had done nothing to damage the relationship.

To put a cherry on top of the sundae, the spring after they returned, I found two of their four children in our backyard, picking apples off our trees. It does not bother me that they took the apples. It would have been nice if someone had mentioned that they wanted some of our apples. More importantly, they could have come by for a quick visit.

In the spring of year twelve, weather permitting, I would load Lynne into her wheelchair for a rolling tour of the neighborhood she walked for years. This provided me with a bit of exercise and Lynne a little sun and fresh air. One afternoon, while I was helping Lynne into the wheelchair on our front step, Nancy was walking by. When she spotted us, more particularly Lynne, she rushed down our driveway with a huge smile on her face.

In her many trips past our house, Nancy had seen me but never saw Lynne. She assumed the worst and did not know how to approach me. With our friendship back on track, we have visited Nancy and her husband on a few occasions, but more importantly, reestablished Lynne's friendship with their dog.

A few days after my mother developed the aspiration pneumonia that ended her life, I told one of our neighbors that this looked like it was the end and that I would have to probably make "the decision" within the next few days. A few days later, abiding by my mother's wishes, I did, in fact, give the order to terminate what had become life support.

The morning after my mother's passing, I told two of the neighbors and asked one of them to spread the word that my mother had passed. She said she would do this, and I thanked her for it. Now, as I write this, is been more than two years since my mother's death, and I have yet to receive a condolence call, card, or any form of expression of sympathy from any of the neighbors except the two whom I told directly. I was raised in a different time and certainly raised better than that. When a neighbor was in trouble or had a death in the family, neighbors were there with food and assistance, because that's the way you are supposed to do it. That's the way we used to do it. I was certainly not expecting a horde of neighbors bearing food and offering assistance. But I certainly was expecting at least a show of sympathy for my loss. My mother's death was their loss too, since she was a neighbor and friend.

I guess I'm too old school or just care too much for people in their time of need or sorrow. But know this—if something were to happen to any of my neighbors, I would be at their door, offering condolence and assistance. Again, that's my way, and I am not going to change based on other's shortsightedness.

I have no scientific proof of this, but I am satisfied that Alzheimer's disease is contagious. Based on my observations, I will leave it to you to determine if you agree. But I am positive that this disease is contagious. As a student of human nature and more than a casual observer of people and their reactions to the unknown or misunderstood, this disease affects more than just the mind of the victim.

In addition to our cast of characters, there is an often interesting group of people. They are all bound by a common thread, which we all will agree cannot be broken. Most of the players in this threepenny opera, while concerned for Lynne, my mother, and myself, have not gone out of their way to help. If anything, they have gone out of their way to stay out of the way. There are the occasional kind words and offers of prayer, but there is no action to back up the concern and supposed desire to help. These people have a name—the Buts. "I would like to help, but . . ." They are always found near the edge of your life, hoping not to be called upon because they are afraid of being inconvenienced or left alone with a sick person.

Most everybody forgets all the promises of help when you need it the most. When they first hear the diagnosis, they are quick to say that they will pray for you, you will be in their thoughts, and those infamous words we have all heard, "If you ever need anything, just let me know." While thoughts and prayers are certainly more than welcome, the assistance that has been offered can become a necessity as you progress further with the disease. The problem is that as you were going through the disease with your loved one, the people who offered assistance have gone into the advanced stage of this communicable form of Alzheimer's disease.

Gone are the friends and relatives who only appear when they need something, and you are their personal ATM or rental center. These leaches still believe they deserve preferential treatment while ignoring your need for assistance. Then they get an attitude when you fail to provide whatever assistance or support they require. They conveniently miss the fact that you are focused on being the best caregiver and cannot be their benefactor any longer.

I wish I could list all the friends and relatives whom my mother, my wife, and I have misplaced because they have this communicable form of Alzheimer's. I know that they were not infected by my mother or my wife, since these friends and relatives could not be found once they heard the diagnosis. I would list these friends and relatives, but it would add several pages, and I am sure someone on this list would remember us enough to come with a hand out, but not to help out. So I guess the moral to this story is that they didn't care enough to start with, so when the chips were down; they ran and hid for fear someone might ask for assistance.

As a caregiver, you have a long list of things to do day in and day out, and if you are like most caregivers, at the end of the day, you still do. Even though I am awake more than twenty hours a day normally, I never seem to make a dent in my list of things to do outside of caring for Lynne. This is another indication that Alzheimer's is contagious. I suffer from a loss of organizational, time management, and decision-making skills.

Most importantly, from a personal standpoint, you begin to forget the good times you and your loved one had over the years.

It becomes increasingly difficult to remember the milestone events, vacations, holiday celebrations, and just the day-to-day things that your relationship was built around that make up the memories of your time together. Instead, your pleasant memories become overrun by what the Alzheimer's has done to you and your loved one. Gone are your plans for the years to come, because they never will. Your thoughts instead are filled with caring for the afflicted and what can you do to help them be safer and more comfortable.

Of course, with all this rhetoric about absent family and disappearing friends, it is possible to have too much of a good thing. Some caregivers have a near-endless list of family and friends who constantly call or stop by to find out how the patient is doing. Frankly, it can be tiresome to have to give bad-news updates all of the time as the patient continues to fail. It is hard to say what the right balance is, as it varies from case to case. But if in doubt, err on the side of being a pest until the caregiver or patient tells you ease up or says, "Don't call us; we'll call you."

When you want to make yourself available to do more than sit and chat, schedule a visit with the caregiver. Don't "if you ever need anything" you way through the offer of assistance just to ease your guilt while not committing yourself. Call the caregiver and say, "I will be coming by next Wednesday at noon; put me to work after we visit for a few minutes."

Touring the AMA

My mother presented with the classic, right-from-the-Alzheimer's-handbook symptoms of short-term memory loss, some confusion, loss of some executive functions, and, of course, an advanced case of denial of having any symptoms, which is the most common symptom—especially among the elderly. After more than a year of asking mom to talk to her doctor about her symptoms, she finally tired of my pestering, and she did mention them to her doctor. The doctor ordered a CT scan, ran blood work, and did a Mini-Mental State Examination (MMSE) to determine if my mother had anything that could mimic the general Alzheimer's symptoms.

When my mother was diagnosed, she did not understand the diagnosis and what it meant for her future. The two reasons for her lack of understanding were simple. She never knew anyone who had the type of problems she was experiencing, and her doctor was not prepared to tell someone they had a fatal disease. Her doctor, who had run all the proper tests for the time based on my mother's complaint of failing memory and some confusion, simply handed her the patient starter pack of Alzheimer's medicine and said, "Take these, and see if it helps your memory."

The doctor was not prepared to deliver the news. She never said the words *Alzheimer's* or *dementia*. It was left to me to understand and explain to my mother what her diagnosis meant, what steps would have to be taken to ensure her safety and care, and the long-term effects of the disease. In my explanation, I did not focus on the fact that this disease would eventually prove to be fatal. I did not tell her that she would eventually become what everybody once called old people—senile. I focused instead on her need in the future to have someone help her more than I was capable of doing.

Lynne presented symptoms that were different from the standard Alzheimer's. In the beginning, her issues just seemed to be same problems most everyone faces as the calendar pages fly by. She was having trouble with the mechanics of reading; her once-perfect handwriting was not so perfect; her vision was suspect (partially due to the lenses in her new glasses being cut incorrectly), and she started to stutter slightly and very occasionally. All of these small glitches just pointed to Lynne simply getting older. In researching these very vague symptoms, I found the term "age-related cognitive decline"—a non-diagnosis if I have ever seen one. In all the reading and researching, the one thing she did not have, according to the norms, was Alzheimer's. She was too young, and the symptoms really did not fit. And most of the fourteen doctors we saw in the five years of searching for a diagnosis did not feel that Lynne's difficulties were any form of dementia.

One possible symptom that I reported to every doctor was Lynne's sleep habits. Before the disease, Lynne slept all over the bed. Many mornings, Ginger and I would be hanging on the edge of our king-size bed after having been chased there because of Lynne's very active sleep. About the time she started with her other symptoms; she began sleeping through the night in the position she took at bedtime. I told each doctor that she slept like she was dead.

Lynne had remarked on a few occasions that her previously perfect handwriting was no longer perfect. Lynne had perfect penmanship—to a point where, while attending a one-room country schoolhouse in Michigan, she was asked to teach the other left-handed students how to write in cursive. I felt, and her primary care physician agreed, that the change in Lynne's handwriting was probably due to early arthritis, and just like most of the working population, she did nearly all of her work on a computer.

Lynne's path along the Alzheimer's diagnosis trail was full of many useless stops throughout the medical community. The diversity of doctors was exceeded only by our desire to find answers to the ever-growing list of questions and symptoms. Admittedly, some of the doctors we chose or were referred to were just grasping at straws. But as time went on, and Lynne kept losing bit by bit, we kept trying.

Lynne was not diagnosed for more than five years after she presented her early symptoms. Why? The doctors were not looking for Alzheimer's in someone in her fifties, and I did not have the information I needed to push for the proper testing. Since we had given the doctors carte blanche, Lynne and I assumed, quite erroneously, that all the possible testing available for her symptoms was being run. We certainly had the doctor bills to prove that they were at least running some tests—just not the right ones. Or maybe they were not interpreting the results correctly. But the fact remained; we had a mystery on our hands.

Our list of doctors included, in no particular order, her primary care doctor, four neurologists in three different practices, two ophthalmologists, two psychiatrists, an allergist, an epidemiologist, a behavioral optometrist, and on it went. Then throw in a cast of nurse practitioners, nurses, physician's assistants, technicians, and office staff members. We ran the gamut of the medical professionals. And of course, no good office visit would be complete without the usual "We need to run some tests," which were often the same tests that had been run before with the same "no reason why" results.

The testing also ran the gamut—EEGs, EKGs, an evoked potential test, blood tests, urine tests, three MRIs, and enough MMSEs to where I could count backward by sevens in my sleep into triple-digit negative numbers. And speaking of sleep, one of the neurologists had Lynne do a sleep study. A quick thousand bucks for a poor night's sleep—and again, no revealing results. She had a glut of neurologic tests run except the one that would give us the answer or at least point us in the right direction to determine what course of treatment was available for returning Lynne to her previous glory.

But the fact remained that we kept searching for the answers with every referral. And each referral just led us to more dead ends and more sleepless nights spent searching the Internet for what we might be dealing with and whom we needed to see to get Lynne the proper testing. Believe me when I say that the Internet is more than just social networking sites, online shopping, and porn. It is an invaluable tool in the search when you have so few solid answers to so many vague questions. It helped us better understand some of the tests, test results, and how to proceed once we received the Alzheimer's diagnosis.

After the overabundance of tests, scans, MMSEs, and all the other feeble attempts by the long list of physicians who all at least made an attempt to answer the questions, Lynne was diagnosed by the fourth neurologist who sent her for a PET scan. I am confident the information that Lynne's primary care doctor supplied as well as the information we brought gave him a fairly good idea of what we were dealing with. He ran but one test and got the answer.

Before we found the doctor who actually diagnosed Lynne, previous doctors felt her symptoms were probably caused by stress or depression. This, according to the drug manufacturers that advertise so heavily, is a very large portion of the population. If Lynne is any example, these complaints of stress and depression could possibly be the early symptoms of Alzheimer's disease. I am not a doctor, but I do know that most of the doctors who examined Lynne wanted to blame depression on her condition. One neurologist even gave Lynne a prescription for an antidepressant before running any tests because "it couldn't hurt."

Mind you, Lynne was in and out of work, so insurance was often not in the picture. When insurance was available, Lynne's problem was always a preexisting condition—even though there was no condition established except vague symptoms for an unknown problem. The bottom line was clear; money was going to become scarcer as time went on, and we were not discovering what Lynne's problem was or what might be causing it. By the time she was finally diagnosed, we had managed to wipe out roughly 75 percent of Lynne's retirement fund and all of our savings.

What did we learn from this medical probing, which was of such little benefit in diagnosing her problem? While in some ways, the results put our minds at ease, the doctors determined Lynne was not suffering from a blood disorder, sleep apnea, STDs, allergies, cancer, Lyme disease, MS, a stroke or series of mini strokes, a blood clot, an eye problem, or a laundry list of things the doctors thought her condition might be, could be, or should be. But it was a cash cow for every doctor we went to see. And now, just like then, with the exception of the fatal disease, she's in perfect health. I am confident that if she had insurance, or we had deeper pockets, the doctors would have started looking for zebras instead of just settling for horses.

Lynne's path to her diagnosis was probably not all that unique. Her symptoms did not conform to the established Alzheimer's diagnostic protocols. We started with her primary care physician, who referred us to the first neurologist. He sent Lynne a ten-page questionnaire a few days prior to her appointment to complete for the office visit. During the visit, he leafed through the questionnaire, asking additional questions along the way. This was followed by a quick physical examination and her first of many MMSEs.

After the questionnaire, interview, and physical examination, the doctor's opinion was that Lynne was suffering from situational stress and that if she changed jobs, the various problems should resolve themselves. We did make it abundantly clear during the interview that Lynne worked in a branch office of hell with the ultimate control freak for a boss. His assessment was that she was unhappy at work, and she should "fire her boss." His care plan was never able to come to fruition, as Lynne was laid off due to budget constraints. Truth be known, her layoff was more of a firing—and justifiably so, due to her increased error rate and inability to take on new projects.

As time marched on, of course, her symptoms only got worse. Lynne's former strong suits—like writing, reading, typing, handwriting, and logic—became the enemy that was telling us things in Lynne's head just were not right. The job change, while certainly an improvement on the employment front, did not alleviate the symptoms.

One of the more unusual specialists we came across was a behavioral optometrist. This field is definitely not mainstream medicine, but it is probably a great alternative to a regular optometrist for patients who are not satisfied with the quality of their vision. With all the research I was doing just trying to get any kind of handle on Lynne's problem, I came across an article that listed her symptoms that seemed written specifically about her. Of the thirteen symptoms listed in the article, Lynne matched eight precisely and three slightly or occasionally. I felt we were on the verge of a breakthrough.

After Lynne and I discussed my discovery of the behavioral optometrist, I immediately went back to the computer to find the nearest one and whether he or she was within driving or flying distance. It did not matter to us how far we needed to travel, since it looked so promising. In the entire Washington-Baltimore region, there was a grand total of two behavioral optometrists. Fortunately, one of the two was only about ten miles from home.

Having spent many hours in the examination rooms with my mother-in-law and her myriad of eye problems, which required a vast array of eye specialists, I felt we had gone back in time when we entered the behavioral optometrist's exam room. The first thing I noticed was the size of the room itself. It was much larger than the exam rooms I was accustomed to. The doctor explained that to get the most accurate results, it was best to use a room that would allow the patient to be twenty feet away from the screen that they were reading from. The examination itself was extremely detailed—much more than just finding the right prescription strength for the glasses he wanted to sell in the front room. He checked the mechanics of her eye movements as he performed the various tests.

After this thorough examination, which lasted well over two hours, the doctor felt that Lynne had, for some unknown reason, suffered a disconnect between her eyes and her brain. We knew it was not due to damage from a blow to the head or the result of a stroke, as those had been tested for and eliminated from the list of possibilities several times before. He recommended that we attend his weekly vision training sessions to try to reestablish the lost connection. We attended these weekly sessions and did the homework for just over one year. Since Lynne had lost yet another job (her last job) shortly after we began our vision training, we were able to train hard every day.

The results were amazing. Within a few months, I hardly ever wore my glasses since I was getting the benefit of the training while demonstrating and guiding Lynne through the various exercises. Lynne's results were not as impressive—actually there was no change in her vision, and her symptoms had continued on the same pace as before.

Memory loss, of course, is everyone's main focus when discussing Alzheimer's disease. After all, AD is touted as a memory disorder. So short-term memory loss is everyone's first Alzheimer's symptom. This is not true in all cases of Alzheimer's disease. Short-term memory loss is the most commonly recognized first symptom. Forgetting names, dates, and personal milestones was not Lynne's apparent first symptom. It took more than seven years after she presented her first symptoms to develop any consistent, identifiable short-term memory loss. This is another example of why Alzheimer's is not a one-size-fits-all disease.

Alzheimer's Facts and Figures

I t is a small but overpopulated world here in Alzheimer's Land. The saddest part is that every sixty-eight seconds, someone receives the diagnosis of Alzheimer's disease. With the current victim population of 5.4 million people in the United States and a caregiver population estimated to exceed 15 million, the possibility of finding people touched by this killer is more than pretty good. And unless things change, it is projected that the victim population will be 16 million by 2050 in the United States. So figuring a ratio of three caregivers for every AD victim, by 2050, the caregiver population will be approaching 50 million. That's approximately 66 million victims and caregivers here in Alzheimer's Land. To give you an idea of what 66 million people represents, I did a quick browse on the Internet. The 2010 census shows the combined population of California and Texas to be 64.6 million people. The numbers are staggering (to say the least) when you think about the lost productivity at work, the goods and services not utilized, and the loss of normalcy in millions of homes from the challenges of Alzheimer's and the burden of caregiving.

You never know who has it, who cares for someone with it, or who wants to learn more about it because they fear the unknown of a disease that affects so many, but is still shrouded in mystery. Even though Alzheimer's was identified over one hundred years ago, the medical community and the drug researchers have made little progress in learning about it. They don't know how or when it begins, if there is a way it can be prevented, or why it affects some but not others. Ideas on how it starts include effects of high blood pressure, high cholesterol, a blow to the head, dental disease, stress, or it may be a new form of diabetes. And like with everything else that people don't understand, they still like to share uninformed opinions about it. I heard a grocery cashier tell a customer that the cause of AD was living in a dusty house. There's also been a lot of speculation that aluminum in our diet is a cause of Alzheimer's disease. I don't know how much proof there is of any of these scenarios, but if any of them are true, we are all doomed!

If you are new to Alzheimer's disease or even an old hand at it, you may not be armed with basics of what this disease is or what to expect. I hope to help you develop a basic understanding of what you and your AD victim are up against.

First, understand that many people do not know what Alzheimer's disease is—and I am not speaking scientifically. Many may say, "Oh, my grandmother had that," or words to that effect. The first misunderstanding I run into time and time again is that dementia is Alzheimer's. But not all dementia is Alzheimer's. Alzheimer's is the leading form of dementia. I also run into the misunderstanding by some that Alzheimer's is curable. As we all find out at the end of the road, it's not.

Alzheimer's is a progressive, degenerative neurologic disease that is always fatal. At present, there is no definitive testing available that can provide an absolute diagnosis of Alzheimer's disease, though there are procedures being tested that do show promise. The only way to get an absolute diagnosis is by autopsy—which, while satisfying to a certain degree, does not help your doctor in care planning or you in your caregiving decisions. So the diagnosis is actually possible or probable Alzheimer's disease. And while we are on the subject of determining Alzheimer's at autopsy, here's a fact from the pages of Alzheimer's history. The patient on whom Dr. Alois Alzheimer performed the autopsy in 1906 was actually, by today's standards, Early Onset. Auguste Deter was fifty-one when she died, having presented strange behavioral symptoms, including short-term memory loss.

Alzheimer's disease is generally referred to as a memory disorder. While technically correct, the term "memory disorder" is very misleading to that point that I feel it influences the way the general public views this disease. "It's no big deal if I forget Aunt Whoever's name or forget where the car keys are." While it is not a "big deal" to have a little memory lapse now and again, the inability to remember could be the very beginning of any number of diseases with no cure and limited treatment options that the patient and caregivers will be involved in for, in some cases, over twenty years. So I will stand on my soapbox and proclaim for all to hear that Alzheimer's is not just a memory disorder. Alzheimer's is more the total destruction of the brain where the loss of memories is of such little importance that not remembering a person's name in the grand scheme of things really is no big deal.

In this "no big deal" Alzheimer's scenario, you will forget every meaningful event in your life, and the lives of the people close to you, and you will forget the people. You have to look forward to forgetting your entire family and every friend, job, vacation, and school you ever attended. You will also forget every meaningful event in your life, like your first crush; first kiss; the prom; your wedding; the birth of your children and grandchildren; getting your driver's license; your first car; your high school graduation; college graduation; your first job; the death of your parents, siblings, or children; events like 9/11; and hundreds of other major and everyday events that made you who you were. Then all of that really does become no big deal, since you eventually will not recognize your face in the mirror anyway.

A few other things this little "no big deal" fatal disease helps you also forget include how to use the bathroom (if you can remember where it is); how to use eating utensils; how to drive; how to use telephones, cell phones, computers, and television remotes; how to find your way home from anywhere; how to find your way through your own home; how to shop and handle money; how to brush your teeth; how to perform simple hygiene acts, like brushing your hair, cutting your nails, and shaving; how to dress correctly, considering the event or weather conditions; how and when to take medication and why; how to swallow, cough, vomit, and blow your nose . . . and the list grows longer with each passing day until you have forgotten how to do everything but breathe. But then that goes away too.

In the early and middle stages of the disease, cognitive changes and losses can happen over months. The victim's mind wanders in and out of the various cognitive levels. One day, the victim may remember; the next, they may not—or someplace in the middle. But when you are dealing with later stages, changes can and do happen—sometimes in minutes. They can be permanent or long-lasting, or the patient might switch back to his or her version of normal after a few hours. It makes the game harder to play when the rules change so frequently and without warning or explanation.

Some erroneously think it is possible to remind, coach, or encourage an Alzheimer's patient to remember how to conform to the rules of the real world. My mother, even though she had been fiercely independent since my father's passing, normally played by the rules; but after the disease took over, and she moved to Happy Valley, she had new rules to live by. The entire time she was at Happy Valley, she was less than a happy camper because they had rules that she did not understand or remember. She could not understand why they at times were upset with her for something that she had done—which, of course, she had forgotten.

A few months into my mother's stay at Happy Valley, I was summoned by the facility director following yet another incident involving my mother. She had once again forgotten their rules. The meeting included the facility director, dementia coordinator, a nurse, and one of the aides. But at no time were we all in the same room at the same time—a shining example of uncoordinated care planning by a professional staff for this scheduled meeting. In this meeting, they asked me to speak to my mother about becoming a "better, more cooperative resident" and convince her not be such a hard case about everything. The long and short of it was they wanted me to get her to fall in line with all the other residents. I think they figured I could order her to play nice.

Obviously, it is hard to teach an old dog new tricks, especially if the old dog can't remember the new trick she was taught yesterday. My mother, like the other Happy Valley residents, was thrust into a strange environment—certainly not a home that they had lived in before. They were all supposed to live by new rules set down by the strangers who were being paid quite handsomely to take care of them. My mother was no different from the rest. She continued to be confused about their rules—the rules she had nothing to do with before she came to what had become her new home by no choice of her own.

For those who are not familiar with the basics of Alzheimer's disease, trying to implant new memories—no matter how simple— is rarely successful, if not impossible. The only thing that is usually accomplished by trying to force new memories is irritating the caregiver and confusing the Alzheimer's victim. It also serves to do nothing more than give you a false sense of success if it works for a few hours after you have introduced the new memory; the patient will just forget it the next day.

But this is Alzheimer's disease, and whatever your victim can or cannot do, the brain that is being destroyed by this disease often will find ways to defy the Alzheimer's code of conduct. While the memories that made them who they were are fading and becoming a hodgepodge of remembrances and voids, the victim's brain must be still trying to develop new memories to fill the emptiness. New memories can rarely be introduced by others, but the AD victim can sometimes still develop new memories on his or her own. Some Alzheimer's victims find a new love and remember the name and physical appearance of their new love but do not remember the spouse they have been with for decades. These new memories are probably the brain looking for comfort or stability.

Milestones are something that only you, the caregiver, will be able to determine. Unlike most fatal diseases, Alzheimer's has no real milestones. The doctor cannot say, "You have Alzheimer's disease, and you've got six months to live." There are two reasons for this. First, there is no definitive diagnosis of Alzheimer's disease, and there are other neurologic conditions that can mimic the symptoms of Alzheimer's. Second, Alzheimer's disease progresses at its own rate in every individual with or without medication.

I warned you that I can and do become preachy about Alzheimer's disease, the caregiving, the treatment, and the currently bleak future. So here goes. We continue to put a Band-Aid on a broken arm. The current treatment plans have been stuck in place for so long to be sure there is something else in the works. While the current treatments are effective for most for a while, there need to be more—and sooner rather than later. There is very little later in any fatal disease, so waiting is really not an option.

Following the tried-and-true treatment plan is the correct way, but at the same time, maybe more thinking outside the box (or the little brown bottle) is long overdue. We have a fatal and very financially, physically, and emotionally costly disease on our hands. And like every disease, we are all at the mercy of the FDA and their vision of the right and wrong approaches to treatment. We need to investigate alternative approaches outside of the FDA. There needs to be more coordination internationally among all parties to arrive at improved protocols to develop the needed treatment plans instead of every pharmaceutical company striking out on its own in the hopes of scoring the potentially multi-billion dollar payday.

There also must be new patent policies for those companies that develop treatments or cures using naturally occurring substances. Naturally occurring substances cannot be patented; therefore, the company that spends the big bucks discovering a naturally occurring substance that treats or cures a disease cannot gain the type of compensation from the end user that the typical laboratory-developed drug can gain the pharmaceutical company that develops and patents it. Without patent protection, every other drug manufacturer can duplicate and sell the product without having the research and development costs.

As I wrote early on, you may detect a deep hatred. A portion of this hatred is, of course, of this insidious disease and what it does to the victims, caregivers, families, and friends. But then there are also the economic costs in medical care, caregiving expenses, and lost productivity. Those who know me might feel the exhaustion from the long hours of caregiving, coming to the end of my wife's battle, had somehow desensitized me and eased my hatred of this disease, since I have resigned myself to the fact that there will be no happy ending to our fairy tale lives together.

This disease lays waste to everything and everybody it comes in contact with, and there is no end in sight. I would be remiss if I did not once again step up on my soapbox to proclaim that Alzheimer's disease, among so many other diseases, will never be cured, and the available treatments will be marginally effective as long as we have the federal government in charge of new drug approval.

This sounds like just another conspiracy theory, but give it some thought for a moment. No person I have shared my theory with who has been touched by this or any other disease, or not, can deny the possibility or probability of this theory. I am not saying that there exists a better treatment or a cure for Alzheimer's or any other disease hiding in a secret file cabinet someplace—but then, who really knows for sure?

Simply put, the Food and Drug Administration (FDA) is responsible for the safety of the food and drugs in the United States. This responsibility includes the approval of new and improved drugs, medical devices, and procedures. The FDA is another branch of the federal government that is responsible for keeping us healthy and safe.

The federal government has another agency that you have probably heard of—the Social Security Administration (SSA). Billions of dollars are distributed to the elderly and disabled by SSA every year in the form of monthly retirement and disability payments. And, of course, SSA is also the home of Medicare, which currently spends $140 billion annually on Alzheimer's disease—and this number is projected to rise to $1.1 trillion by 2050.

So what do these two offices of the federal government have to do with each other, and why will there never be a cure for so many life-ending diseases? It is a very simple math problem. Since Social Security is drowning in red ink—and will be for the foreseeable future—SSA needs a way to control the amount of money paid out. What better way to control the outflow of cash than to have the recipients of benefits taken off the books? With over 5.4 million Alzheimer's victims, most receiving benefits from SSA, how much more money would be spent by the federal government if there were suddenly a cure for Alzheimer's? Adding an untold number of years of monthly retirement benefit payments and additional Medicare payments for the 5.4 million former AD victims would certainly push SSA over the edge. Based on the average $1,200 monthly SSA retirement check, keeping five million now-recovered AD patients on the books for ten additional years would mean approximately $800 billion in additional SSA retirement payments alone.

Does the federal government have a vested interest in not allowing cures or improved treatments to be approved? The FDA makes the drug companies jump through endless numbers of bureaucratic hoops by tying up the approval process for literally years—sometimes for drugs that have been previously approved for other diseases. At the same time, the FDA rushes to market treatments and cures for nonfatal diseases and vanity drugs—some with the possibility of extreme side effects.

I know—at least; I hope—that the FDA does have our best interests in mind. But somehow, the approval process has to be sped up—not just for Alzheimer's, but all fatal diseases. I know this sounds very idealistic, but maybe the FDA should examine the possible side effects of death and the need for long-term care. Shouldn't the disease victim decide how much he or she is willing to risk with drug side effects versus facing certain death or needing long-term care?

———————

Having seen firsthand and heard so many stories from other caregivers, as well as health care professionals, I firmly believe the health care system is not able to work with cognitively challenged patients and their families consistently and effectively. Diseases like Alzheimer's destroy the patient's ability to communicate effectively, so emergent problems can quickly become major problems.

To be blunt, why should doctors or their staff members become emotionally invested in a dying patient? For some doctors, an AD patient is just an excellent profit center—a few minutes in the office, a quick prescription refill, and then out the door. All that is left is filing the insurance. I know there are many who care, but of the two neurology practices we visited after Lynne was diagnosed, only one has taken time to talk about the changes in Lynne, ask how I am doing, bring us up to speed on the current research, and originate Lynne's entry into hospice.

Support for patients and their caregivers must first involve education about the disease as well as all available services and programs. I have seen too many doctors in action, and it is seldom that the doctor gives you important information in writing. They talk, you listen, you go home, and you forget everything that was said and why. It would be very beneficial for, say, a neurologist who has just delivered the Alzheimer's diagnosis to have information written in plain English (or the appropriate language) informing the patient and the patient's family of what is coming and especially what can or cannot be done—an "Introduction to Alzheimer's" if you will.

The information is out there, but there needs to be a standardized, up-to-date handbook available for the patients and families so they can understand the basics of the disease. Doctors spend years studying to become doctors. They should not expect the layperson to have ready access to the answers to the rush of questions regarding the diagnosis and patient support, especially moments after receiving the diagnosis of a fatal disease. In an ideal world, the doctor would deliver the bad news to the victim and the family, and before they left the office, they would be handed this introduction to Alzheimer's.

The victim, family, and caregivers should not have to spend valuable time reinventing the wheel, searching for information on the Internet (provided they have access and know-how) that may or may not be valid, up-to-date, or safe. I am fortunate that I had the time to develop a battle plan (albeit an ever-changing one) while Lynne was still capable and cognizant enough to bear with me while I learned.

As the population ages, Alzheimer's disease will be a growing concern for millions more. As the sole caregiver for my mother and my wife, I am concerned with the number of people who just don't understand or have access to information about what this disease is really all about. Even experienced caregivers have limited information about the disease and programs that are available to assist in the seemingly never-ending battle. While the government has taken a few steps to increase its presence in the lives of those with the disease by throwing a few million more bucks into the pot, there must be more real information available so the public will stop just thinking that Grandma is just getting old and acting odd when, with proper education, families can get the potential Alzheimer's victim the proper medical care, which may buy them a few more quality years. And in Lynne's case, "Grandma" was in her early fifties when this "old folk's disease" started showing its first very discrete symptoms.

Education alone is not going to cure the disease or develop better treatment plans, but it is so necessary in the ongoing fight. I see breast cancer ads on television almost daily. Maybe Alzheimer's education should take the same direction. My experience with the Alzheimer's Association has always been good, but I also find it to be lacking. This disease is still shrouded in mystery for the medical community, drug companies, caregivers, and, of course, the victims. Maybe it's time to shed more light on the subject and make the people not yet directly affected aware of more details concerning the number one form of dementia, what everyone is dealing with who has Alzheimer's in their family, and most importantly, what is in store for them should this very silent killer continue unabated. As the population ages, the number of Alzheimer's victims will continue to rise. As I write this, Alzheimer's disease is the only disease in the top-ten causes of death that is still on the increase and has no cure or means of prevention.

———————

The list of ways to avoid or delay the onset of Alzheimer's is long and getting longer, depending on who's funding these studies we are always hearing about. Keep your brain active; do things that will exercise your brain, like crossword or Sudoku puzzles; get physical exercise; drink X cups of coffee; drink X glasses of wine; take vitamins; eat this, but don't eat that . . . and the list just keeps growing. I am not saying any or all the above are effective or ineffective in combating Alzheimer's or any other disease. What I am here to tell you is that, between my two Alzheimer's patients, they have consumed enough coffee to fill the Pentagon, did countless crossword and logic puzzles, could put together a ten thousand piece jigsaw puzzle effortlessly, and enjoyed a vigorous walk for thirty to sixty minutes nearly every day for over thirty years. So what does "do this, don't do this, eat this, exercise this, ad infinitum" really mean?

Your chances of developing this disease are most likely not controlled by your food consumption and exercise habits as much as your genes and what they have to say about your future. I am not for one second saying that physical and mental exercise and proper nutrition are not good for you, but these factors are probably not really going to help you avoid Alzheimer's—or most any other medical condition—if it's in your genes.

But here is something to scratch your head over. Our little slice of Fairfax seems to be a dementia cluster. Five houses side-by-side feature five dementia victims—vascular dementia, Alzheimer's, no apparent neurologic deficits, Parkinson's and Early Onset Alzheimer's, and Alzheimer's, respectively. So maybe it's not what you eat or drink or how much physical and mental exercise you get. Maybe it's environmental.

———

According to the Alzheimer's Association, there are seven stages of Alzheimer's disease. (You will find this list at *www.alz.org* and in the back of my book.) For most people, these stages are simply general warning signs. But for others these stages can be horrifying previews of the unknown coming attractions.

Shortly after my mother was diagnosed, Lynne and I attended some Alzheimer's Association support group meetings. I do recommend that you try to attend a few sessions. They can provide a strong dose of reality when you listen to the other caregivers and their stories; since these meetings have no AD patients in the audience, caregivers can speak freely. The group usually meets once a month and costs you nothing. And depending on the area, there can be many meeting times and locations to choose from. Sometimes attending a meeting or two can help you gain valuable insight on this disease and your rapidly approaching new responsibilities.

Some of the attendees and their stories will amaze, some will confuse, but everybody has one thing in common. You are all in a fleet of caregiving boats bobbing around in the Alzheimer's ocean. All of these little caregiving boats have another thing in common; they are all going to sink—just at different rates.

Customarily, the moderator will open with any news from the world of Alzheimer's and then will go around the room, asking each person to share because everybody in this sinking fleet is willing to learn, willing to share, or just wants to communicate with another adult on an adult level. Some of these experiences may help you or someone else in attendance. You can also gain some insight into how the various caregivers interpret the stages of their AD victim.

Our monthly support group meetings were held in a library meeting room several miles from our home. I had spoken with the group moderator, and she asked that we attend her group because she felt I had the type of personality that could bring something to her group. The group was small—about twelve people. Most had been in the group for a while.

At our first meeting, when we did the sharing portion, a man and his daughter (also first-timers) told the group of their wife/mother, who was the AD victim. Based on the husband's age, I made the assumption that his wife was Early Onset. The husband was armed with several folders and notebooks detailing the *what, why,* and *when* of how his wife was handling her disease. He had a spreadsheet with each her daily activities, and in his opinion, what stage she was at with each activity. He was quick to point out that his wife did not follow the proper order in doing many of her regular activities (also known as "his way"). He further went on to state numerous times that he retired on March 18 so he could stay at home to care for his wife. He was approaching his caregiving duties in a very organized, businesslike manner with all the proper documentation. Frankly, he came across as a frustrated businessman with a product that was not performing up to his specifications.

The daughter, on the other hand, was both emotionally and physically involved in her mother's care. She was in her thirties and living at home so she could help out. Every workday, she would leave her job at lunch time and drive home to help her mother. I do not know the whole situation, but it seems to me that Mr. "I retired on March 18 to care for my wife" could have taken the lunch shift so their daughter wouldn't have to leave work, drive forty-five minutes one way, check on and help her mother, and then return to finish her workday. And I know the type of drive it was, as her work location was just a few blocks from our home, and the family lived near the library where we were meeting.

At another support group visit, during the sharing portion, one of the attendees had a very typical sad story and the all-too-frequent realization of what comes at the end of the caregiver's job. "Emily" was helping the staff of an Alzheimer's facility care for her eighty-year-old mother, and like so many caregivers, she was burning the candle at both ends, trying to take care of her job and her family during the day and helping care for her mother at the facility at night.

Every evening after work, Emily would go to visit with her mother, feed her, bathe her, and get her ready for bed. One evening, Emily was asked to attend a care planning meeting at the facility. A staff member took over the responsibilities of the very dutiful daughter for that evening. While readying Mom for bed, somehow Mom's dentures became lost. The facility director apologized fully and told the daughter that it was apparently their fault, so they would cover the cost of the replacement dentures and any other fees involved. In my mind, this is a happy ending, and I would be trotting my loved one to the dentist to get the replacement dentures. While the process would have probably been exciting, to say the least, it would be the end of the story.

I had never met Emily before that night. Maybe she just had too much on her plate, and it was affecting her thought process. First she blamed herself for not being there for her mother. In fact, she was there for her mother because she was in the care planning meeting with the staff. Her big concern was not financial, since the facility was handling that. Emily was in a panic since she would have to find a dentist who would be able to handle an Alzheimer's patient. But that was a concern; of course, that was not the problem. The problem was that because her mother's dentures were missing, "It makes her look so old." And with that, the tears started flowing, and she repeated multiple times, "It makes her look so old. It makes her look so old."

Like I said, I did not know this woman, having only met for the first time that night. I was also confident that I had never met her mother. But it seems to me that when you have to put your eighty-year-old mother into an Alzheimer's facility, she has pretty much reached the "old" category. The fact that Mom was looking so old was not the real issue. Emily was probably finally facing her mother's mortality. Being a caregiver or being on the sidelines while you watch your loved one fade away is a stressful job.

At every meeting we attended was one of the regulars, "Karen," whose mother was in an Alzheimer's facility. She had obviously been with the group for some time based on the familiarity other regulars had with her situation. It seems that Mom was in one of the nicer facilities in the Northern Virginia area, and Karen would visit Mom every day without fail and had for a few years.

While Karen went to see Mom every day after driving several miles to get to the facility, she also drove past her sister's house. Her sister, "Diane," lived less than three blocks from Mom's Alzheimer's facility and had never once entered the facility to visit her mother. It was not because they had a longstanding feud. Diane did not want to see Mom in her failing state. But that did not stop her from constantly calling Karen to complain about how poorly Mom was being cared for based on Diane's occasional telephone calls to the facility. A brother living in Atlanta who came to visit Mom once or twice a year was also complaining to Karen because of what Diane was saying about their mother's care.

The moral of this confusing story is that everybody's got an opinion. Some opinions have a basis. Some are unfounded, but they all have one thing in common—they should be kept to the author unless there is a true basis for concern because of personal knowledge of the situation. But if you have a family, be prepared for criticism of your caregiving techniques, whether you are doing it in your own home or assisting the staff at a facility.

At an Early Onset support group meeting, one woman remarked that her husband, the AD victim, seldom wanted to have sex. And it had been that way for well over a year. A second woman responded sadly that her husband was quite the opposite—wanting to have sex multiple times every day since his short term memory loss did not allow him the pleasure of remembering having had sex recently. I was not in attendance at this particular support group meeting, but I feel I would have responded with, "I think there's room for compromise to alleviate the suffering of these two women!" It's just a thought.

Remember the fairy tale opening? I have read much about this disease and have seen most every made-for-television production about Alzheimer's. These authors and script writers certainly must be residents of Fantasyland. Mom or Dad is so quick to respond positively to everything asked of him or her by the calm, cool, and collected team of caregivers. The Alzheimer's victim welcomes a tour of the assisted living facility and then volunteers to move in so he or she won't be a bother. The AD facility shows scores of demented residents enjoying life as if they haven't a care in the world. Each and every one of the dying, demented patients goes ever so peacefully into the next world. Other caregivers, professional and nonprofessional, and I agree—what a bunch of crap! It may be that way for some, but I have not spoken to one caregiver who has experienced dementia in Fantasyland. And nobody else I have talked with has met any other caregiver who reports having the ideal, cooperative, and still functioning AD victim either.

Let me put a little real world perspective on the normal struggles of caring for your AD loved one who just refused medicine, cursed you out for whatever you thought you did right, or the thousands of problems, hiccups, or missteps that happen every day in this minefield of caregiving. I have been around a fair amount of dementia patients and witnessed a wide variety of moods, antics, and responses to authority.

Stacy, one the nurses from hospice, reminded me of the adage, "I cried because I had no shoes until I met a man that had no feet." One of Stacy's previous positions was as a nurse at a dementia facility that was the home to survivors of the Holocaust. Imagine the horror of having uniformed medical staff escorting you into a shower stall when your only clear memories date back to Nazi Germany, where you watched your family and friends being tortured and killed. So you think you have it bad? Walk a mile—not in Fantasyland, but in the real world.

The mission we caregivers have accepted, whether we like it or not, is full of loss and disappointment. The key to staying in the game and not falling into depression (at least for me) is realizing that someday, the battle my loved ones fight every day will hopefully end peacefully. I firmly believe that there is a reward for them in a place called Heaven for having lived their lives in a good way. I believe that once they have shuffled off this mortal coil; they will become whole again. I also believe that Lynne, at her young age for this disease, could have been instrumental in finding a better treatment or a cure by her participation in the two clinical trials at Georgetown.

Planning for the
Present and the Future

Just when you think this caregiving job is only about feeding, dressing, and butt-wiping, you probably will become involved with all the paperwork that is, unfortunately, part of long-term care and death. In general, it can be broken down into three broad categories: legal, financial, and daily responsibilities. And even though these are broad categories, they can and do overlap. So spend time on the Internet, spend time in the library, or do the right thing and consult with an attorney who specializes in elder law, estates, and the like. An attorney can and most likely will cost you money, but making a mistake in the paperwork or the distribution of assets could cost you a whole lot more in the long run.

If you are responsible for the maintenance and distribution of assets, it is important to know what you are dealing with—but more importantly, how to deal with it. I had the luxury of being able to sort through my inheritance before my mother's death. Since I was the sole beneficiary of her estate, I stood very little chance of having my inheritance challenged. You may not have these luxuries of time and no competition, so get it all on paper sooner rather than later, and let the games begin. You may be fighting a war on multiple fronts if you have a lot of value in the estate and a large group of interested family members. Also be prepared for people to say things like, "She said she wanted me to have that when she died." Maybe so, but if it is not in writing, it should be left up to the executor of the estate to decide what to do.

Having a qualified attorney onboard is especially important if fighting over assets becomes a battle of the wills (no pun intended). The time to act is before the victim is incapacitated or has passed away. But know this, when you become responsible for your parent's financials, because of paranoia that is inherent in dementia, there will likely be trust issues—especially if your parent doesn't remember you.

If you and your loved one have the type of relationship in which you do your job and they do theirs, don't be surprised when something comes up that was formerly the AD victim's job. Learning about your partner's usual responsibilities before the dementia takes over may be a bit overwhelming at first, but it is better to have the information, skills, and knowledge before you need it. And I am not just talking about paying the bills or getting the car fixed. I am talking about absolutely everything—cooking, banking, cleaning, filing taxes, and the list of everyday responsibilities that could fill several pages. But I think you understand what I mean.

As the caregiver, you carry the load. You will be both parts of the partnership. And the sooner you understand your partner's responsibilities, the better off you will be. Learning the new responsibilities sooner will give you time to develop a system that will lead to a successful future of caregiving and managing all of the responsibilities that you both used to share.

But also know this—the longer you wait to start taking over these responsibilities, the more resistance you likely will run into. Instead of approaching it with a proactive, "I'm helping you" attitude, you end up with a defensive, "I'm not trying to take anything away from you" attitude. You also run into the situation in which the AD victim could feel like you're treating him or her like a child or undermining their authority.

So the bottom line is this—the sooner the better in taking over all of the jobs for your partnership so you will hopefully reduce the possibility of objections being raised. That is not to say that sometime in the future, you will not run into an "I used to do that; why are you doing it now?" situation. The longer you have been taking care of your loved one's responsibilities, the more likely he or she won't ask, "Why you and not me?" because it will seem that you have always done them. Be prepared for it, and handle it the best you can without losing your cool.

Family friends Carl and Donna had the usual relationship in which he handled all the home repairs on their hundred-year-old farmhouse. Carl had an extensive network of suppliers to help him with cheaper-priced materials and buddies who would do the work. Donna knew few of these people. When Carl died, the old farmhouse that was held together with discounted materials installed by Carl's friends began to need major work. Donna faced the possibility of spending a large portion of her retirement to repair the house or sell it. She sold it at a drastically reduced price since the house needed a lot of work.

It has been said that money makes the world go round, is the root of all evil, and can't buy happiness, but it is certainly going to be the subject of a lot of conversations and probably battles between the caregiver, the AD victim, and family members who always want what's best for the victim—until they find out they have been left out of the will.

For some people, the bank is the end-all and be-all of investments. Savings accounts and CDs are often the only investment vehicles they know and trust. Expect resistance if you broach the subject of using your AD victim's money to buy stocks, bonds, mutual funds, and the like. This may sound sneaky, but use your best judgment if you decide to up the ante on their investments without their knowledge. But remember when dealing with your parent's money that it is still their money, so keep the risk as low as possible. You certainly don't want to have to tell your loved one that you lost their life savings on a "sure thing" bad investment.

I have a reputation of knowing a bit about money and investing, but that's the subject of a whole different book for a whole different time. What I do know about money in this end-of-life scenario is that in no uncertain terms, unless you are skilled in handling investments, you should seek professional help for your loved one's money while at the same time covering your butt. Any error in the financials can cost you big-time. Telling attorneys and the IRS that you didn't know or you didn't understand isn't going to save you. "The Internet said . . ." isn't much of a defense either. So the time to get your ducks in a row is sooner rather than later for the obvious reason—your loved one is suffering from a progressive, degenerative disease with a timetable of its own.

As I said, I have a good reputation when it comes to money and investments. But I also have a reputation of knowing when to say when. So with all this being said, in 2010, I decided to turn the bulk of our investments over to a money manager with one of the big-name Wall Street firms. I was no longer able to watch the market and do the required research, since Lynne needed me more, and, of course, I still had the daily non-caregiver responsibilities to manage. I still have my hand in the game with a small portfolio I can still manage in the little bit of spare time I can find, but the largest portion is being well cared for while I am in caregiver mode.

With all things involving your victim's finances, especially when caring for a parent, there will be the professionals or institutions that have advised your parent before you had to step in and start making the decisions. This is one of the battles that you will surely face because Mom and Dad have been dealing with these people, or their parents, for decades. The question of their qualifications is not a battle that you can dictate the terms of. It may eventually come to having to put your foot down and probably hurt some feelings, since you are now the person responsible for the finances of your loved one.

Your parent may say, "We've used Cousin Fred for our investments for years" or "Joe, our minister's son, wrote our wills fifteen or twenty years ago." While these people may be highly qualified to do the job, it is incumbent upon you as the caregiver and the responsible party to check the credentials of these people. Get all of the paperwork, statements, and any other documents pertaining to the financials. If you are confused, find a qualified third party to examine the documents, and have him or her explain the details of what you are now responsible for and if there are any better options. It may cost you a few bucks, but it may be the cheapest money you have ever spent.

It is important to find individuals or organizations that are truly qualified to assist you with investments, estates, and the day-to-day financial needs of the person you are caring for. Day-to-day banking is pretty simple, but it is still necessary to sit down and talk with the banker with all the proper documentation in hand and discuss the situation. Conducting bank business is often little more than just signing the checks to pay the bills after you have convinced your cognitively challenged person that you are not going to make off with his or her money. Remember that the money is your loved one's money, not yours to spend freely, even if your cognitively challenged loved one says, "What's mine is yours." The tough part comes when dealing with the end-of-life scenario and all the legal and financial aspects of it. And for those ancient wills—things change over the years with regard to estate law, the value in the estate, and the list of beneficiaries.

My best advice, which my mother, my wife, and I all employed, is to find an attorney who specializes in estate and/or elder law and practices in your state, since he or she will likely have better knowledge of the laws and how they apply to your specific situation. Believe me, there is a raft of paperwork involved in this part of caregiving, and while I know there is a vast array of online legal websites and public libraries full of information, sometimes interpreting the legalese could send you down the wrong path. Remember, laws vary from state to state, and using the paperwork drawn up in one state may not work in another. The bottom line is to protect all interested parties with the proper paperwork as soon as possible so everybody understands—at least at that point in time.

Unfortunately, in order to protect your loved one, yourself, and all interested parties, you may have to shell out a few bucks to have a qualified professional in your corner. I am not saying you are not qualified to do what's best. But you really have to be sure. You cannot erase in error because you thought you understood something on the Internet or from a magazine article about estate planning. The list of interested parties in your errors or misunderstandings includes, of course, the IRS and every relative you haven't seen in a dozen years. But just like a vulture, these parties start circling when they smell money. It is said that it takes money to make money. I'm here to tell you that you need to spend money to keep from losing the money, or have it tied up for years defending the estate through a messy challenge to the will. This will cost more money—especially if you lose.

One of my favorite examples of questionable professional assistance is from a close friend of the family. This is a great example of how the trusted professional who has always been there for your loved one may not always be your best option.

"John" lost his mother some years ago. John's mother had a well-respected, highly qualified estate attorney draw up all the documents inherent in getting old and preparing for the end, which included the transfer of her home to John. John's mother, "Leslie," a widow, had lived in her home for many years and was still living there upon her death.

Following Leslie's death, when tax time rolled around, John gathered up all of the paperwork, including the HUD-1 (real estate settlement form) from the sale of Leslie's house. He went to "Phil," the CPA whom Leslie had used for over twenty years, to prepare the taxes. John felt that Phil knew his business since Phil had been a CPA for many years, Leslie had always spoken well of him, and most importantly, Leslie had never been audited. After making sure all the receipts were accounted for, John told Phil to contact the estate attorney about the transfer of the house. John told Phil that the attorney had done something concerning Leslie's house that would possibly decrease John's tax liability, but he did not recall what it was, since it happened several years prior, and John was not really involved with Leslie's estate planning process.

After Phil crunched the numbers, John's federal and state tax liability was over $70,000. John spoke with the estate attorney who drew up Leslie's papers regarding the huge tax bite. John remembered that the attorney had indicated there would likely be taxes due, but he did not remember that the amount owed would be that much. The attorney disagreed with Phil's results and put John in touch with another CPA, "Dan," to double-check Phil's numbers, armed with all of the information concerning the property transfer. Dan and the estate attorney talked to each other, as John had suggested to Phil, and the bottom line was that the new tax liability was zero. It seems that Phil had not contacted the attorney about the details of the property transfer, so he had no knowledge of how to save John thousands of dollars.

My advice is for you to talk to the professionals who know how the laws apply to you and your loved one. It may not work out as well for you as it did for John, but it did save him $70,000, which I think we can all agree is more beneficial to him than to the tax man. In order to have the paperwork drawn up for Leslie, the fee from the attorney was less than $5,000. If you are a bottom-line sort of person like I am, it looks like John's ahead seventy grand because of Leslie's five grand investment in doing the right thing.

Before you start selling estates, transferring assets, and generally getting your financial house in order, do some research. It helps to become familiar with the terms and some of the possible options available before selecting qualified professionals to help you wade through the shark-infested waters of finance. Talk to people who have been there, quiz the Internet, and read the various financial publications regarding the financial issues that are involved while you are caring for your eventually mentally challenged individual. As much as we don't like to talk about a loved one's eventual demise, you have to know how it will affect your financial situation so you can make any possible adjustments. It sounds cold, but you really need to know how your loved one's death with affect your financial future.

Remember Donna from the hundred-year-old farmhouse? With the money from the sale of the house and her retirement savings, Donna sought out a financial advisor to handle her money—and handle it he did. While her advisor never embezzled any of her funds, he did seem to have an inordinate amount of trades that equaled high commissions. Most of his trades were good trades, but there were just so many that the amount of commissions she paid affected her bottom line.

Ignoring the advice of her close friends to drop this money manager, Donna stayed with him until he went on vacation one day, never to return. This vacation seemed to coincide with the authorities beginning an investigation in his business practices. She and other investors who trusted this man were out many thousands of dollars because of the frequent trades and his ability to smooth the ruffled feathers of his many retired clients with slick talk and a smile. So do your homework on any professional before you start funding any new investment account.

———— ∿∿∘◦◦◦◦∿∿ ————

When or if you become the responsible party for the utilities of your AD victim's home, determine what the ground rules are concerning each utility company. I had never become the responsible party or shared responsibility on my mother's utilities since I figured the that power of attorney was sufficient to conduct any business over and above paying the monthly bills, which I had been doing for her for several years.

After my mother moved to Happy Valley, I left the utilities on since I would be working on the house and wanted to leave lights on timers so the house would not look vacant. I also wanted to keep the heat on to keep the pipes from freezing. After a few months, I did have the telephone disconnected since the only calls she was receiving were from charities wanting her annual pledge.

When we disconnected the telephone, we stretched the truth a bit. I called the telephone company, explained that my mother wanted to disconnect her telephone service since she was no longer living in her home because of advancing dementia, and she was not able to live alone any longer. When the customer service representative asked to speak with Mrs. Tutor, I put Lynne on the telephone. With a slight stutter in her voice, she identified herself as Mrs. Tutor and said she wanted to stop her telephone service, since she had moved. With that, Lynne handed the telephone back to me, and I concluded the stopping of my mother's telephone service.

When my mother's house was finally sold and settled, I called the various utilities to shut off their services. The water and electricity were simple. The water department took my word for my relationship to my mother and the circumstances (small-town government at its finest). The water was shut off within minutes of my call. The electric service was nearly as simple. I had to fax the company a copy of the power of attorney, and the electricity was terminated on the Monday following my Friday afternoon call.

The gas company proved to be a formidable adversary prepared to battle to keep my mother's account from ever being closed. My request to shut off the gas, since my mother was no longer the owner of the property, was answered with, "She has to come to the office and shut it off in person." Even with a legally executed power of attorney in hand, I could not take any action on her account. I explained that she was living in an Alzheimer's facility but at the time was in the ICU at the hospital, so her ability to appear at their office was not feasible. Their reason puzzled me. They would not honor the power of attorney since it had not been drawn up or executed in the District of Columbia, their headquarters location. Even with my offer of notarized documentation backing my claim of her dementia and ICU hospitalization, they still would not allow me to take any action regarding her account. After several sometimes heated telephone calls over the next two weeks, I suddenly received the final bill from the gas company. Being the inquisitive type, I called and asked what happened, hoping that my tenacity had finally won the day. The new owner had simply opened a new account, which I guess took precedence over my requests.

We have established that caregiving is seldom easy, and there will always be unforeseen problems. After all of the utilities had been shut off and the final bills paid in full, somehow all of them had been overpaid, and I received refund checks. So one day when Lynne and I were out running a few errands, we stopped by the big, big bank to deposit these checks. And of course, we had a problem. The eighteen-dollar refund check from the water department was made out to Mrs. Grady L. Tutor. The big, big bank would not honor the check since it had no record with the name Grady. I explained to the branch manager that there would be no record since my father had died forty-five years earlier. The "Mrs." was simply added to the account following his death so my mother would have her name on the account and would not have to pay a deposit for opening a new account. The explanation fell on deaf ears; they would not honor the check.

I know that I could have contacted the water department to have them reissue the check in my name. But it was not the amount of the check; it was the principal. I was not going to let the big, big bank push me around. I asked the manager to reconsider, and without hesitation, he said no. So I made him a counteroffer. It seems I had a fairly high balance in my accounts, having recently deposited the proceeds from the sale of my mother's house. I ask him to deposit the eighteen-dollar check out of the goodness of his heart, or I could get a cashier's check for the six-figure balance of my various accounts. It was his choice. Following the deposit, I thanked him for making the right choice. I also told him, "I'm an Alzheimer's caregiver, so don't piss me off—I'm already on the edge."

—⁓•◦ℯ✿◦ℯ◦ℯ◦◦⁓—

Obviously, you want or need to keep track of your caregiving expenses for tax purposes. But if your loved one receives Social Security Disability benefits, somebody, likely you, will be designated as their representative payee. But before you go out spending your loved one's check on things not for them and their care, remember two things. Your loved one's money is to be spent on him or her, and every year, you will have to show SSA how the money was spent on your AD victim and how any money left over was saved.

———∿∾∿∾∾∿———

Since you know that Alzheimer's is terminal, get the funeral arrangements made after you have come to grips with the reality of the situation. Funerals are not cheap, and the funeral homes usually make their money when the family isn't thinking straight. Also, if you are going to write your loved one's obituary, do it sooner rather than later. We are all swept up in the emotion of the pending loss of a loved one, so work on the funeral arrangements and the obit when you are able to do it rationally. I made Lynne's funeral arrangements about a month after we buried my mother. There was a high-value, limited-time coupon, so I took advantage. The obit took me about two years and dozens of drafts to write.

———∿∾∿∾∾∿———

As the disease begins taking more and more of your victim, you are faced with taking more from them also. Diminished cognition makes AD victims a possible danger to themselves and others. So you will be faced with taking away the freedoms that your parents have enjoyed since before you were born or your spouse, sibling, or child since they reached their teen years. This will be tough on both of you, but it must be done, no matter how painful. Your options are extremely limited, and while you wish to avoid hurting your loved one's feelings or starting a fight, taking away driving privileges and not allowing unaccompanied walks around the neighborhood, shopping, or doing previously safe tasks around the house is necessary to ensure the safety of the AD victim, the general public, and you.

One of the greatest losses of freedom for most AD victims is suffering the loss of the car. The car represents freedom, and more importantly, the way to escape your control that will allow them to live a normal life once again. The loss of driving privileges for any adult is a personal insult because everyone says he or she is a good driver with a spotless record and never as much as a parking ticket. And the older the driver, with all of those years of driving experience, the greater the battle will be for control of the keys.

When making the decision about taking away the AD victim's driving privileges, remember what a family friend told me—"If Hazel has an accident where someone is killed, she won't remember it, but you will. And you have a long time to live with the guilt of not parking her."

In conversations with other caregivers or family members, the battle for the control of the car is often where dementia victims will have a resurgence of the executive reasoning skills that all thought were lost. Somehow, no matter how poor your loved one's cognitive skills have become, he or she knows that you will be taking away the driving privileges. Your cognitively challenged loved one will find a way to somehow have replacement keys hidden, have someone replace or repair the equipment that you have removed or disabled, or just borrow a car from a friend who knows you are crazy for even thinking your loved one has Alzheimer's disease.

The risk of having a person with limited cognitive skills behind the wheel isn't just the accident waiting to happen. Even though the victim may have lived in his or her town or even neighborhood for years or decades, they can still get lost. Familiar landmarks from years ago change or disappear, or unexpected detours because of construction or accidents can put them in unfamiliar places.

When my mother's driver's license was about to expire, she was still recovering from her broken hip. While the broken hip was unfortunate, it provided a perfect roadblock that prevented my mother from renewing her driver's license before it expired. Renewing an expired license in Virginia requires that the applicant bring a birth certificate along with the renewal application. I used this to my advantage, especially after her birth certificate had magically disappeared while she was at rehab. In order to get a replacement from North Carolina, I told her that, according to the state archives website, we would have to wait at least six to eight weeks. Using various delaying techniques, including her van not being able to start (for some unexplained reason), I was able to delay her trip to the DMV for several months.

When I could delay her no longer, the DMV and the Commonwealth of Virginia slammed the door on my mother's driving when she could not pass the vision test. Even though we could have gotten a waiver from her ophthalmologist, what she didn't know certainly would not hurt her or the general public. The whole ordeal frustrated her greatly, but it was okay, since it kept her off the road—and I wasn't the bad guy, which is always a good thing. My mother's van started immediately after she moved to Happy Valley when I had the opportunity to reinstall the battery. I took no chances because you don't need a driver's license to drive.

On the other hand, Lynne's driving privileges were halted when she recognized that she was having some difficulties driving at night, especially in the rain. She told me it was getting progressively more difficult to distinguish the tail lights on the cars from the street lights. So Lynne took herself out of the driver's seat before any real symptoms of the AD presented.

The key to successful caregiving is always having a backup plan for your well-thought-out, can't-possibly-fail plan. We all have learned or will learn that no matter how well you anticipate and plan for the contingencies, Alzheimer's or something will get in the way.

I knew I was not going to be able to maintain a presence in two houses, caring for my two AD victims for much longer. So as mayor of Realityville, I needed to develop and execute a plan to care for Mom and Lynne that would not kill me in the process. I had to develop and implement a well-thought-out plan sooner rather than later to hopefully ease the transition from the "old, not working" way to the "what's best for all" way. I had to be in both houses to be constantly aware of both of my loved one's conditions, needs, and situations. I usually called or visited my mother, especially at mealtimes, to make sure she was eating and not falling asleep while cooking or forgetting to turn off the stove.

My mother had been living "independently" for over forty years, and like most Alzheimer's victims, she knew she didn't need any help—except for the ten times a day I got telephone calls to come help. I knew that my mother did not want to leave her museum of a house. She told me many times she did not want strangers living with her, and for some strange reason, she did not want to go into a nursing home or any other facility. I know part of her resistance to nursing homes and assisted living was remembering the less than ideal conditions of the nursing home that she had to put my grandmother in twenty-eight years prior.

Our plan was to move my mother into our house, but it was going to require some serious upgrades, since the part of the house she would be living in was built in the 1950s with narrow halls and doorways and a very tiny bathroom. Of course, anti-wandering equipment also had to be added. Since we did not have the money to make all of the modifications and I couldn't borrow it from my mother, the coordinator at Happy Valley, Lynne, and I hatched a somewhat devious plan to get my mother into the nearby facility and let the staff handle it from there. While she was at Happy Valley, I would clean out, clean up, and make repairs to her house, sell it, make the changes to my house, and move her in with us. I was concerned that, with the close proximity of her house, we might have problems if she remembered that the house two doors up the street was where she used to live. But we had no choice but to take the risk and fight that fire later.

Our great plan began to come together in October 2007. We got my mother into Happy Valley and took off—or as they call it in the assisted living business, "dump and run." She was, in a word, *pissed!* My plan was sound, and step one was complete. Step two went into motion with the two girls who had been doing the weekly cleaning of my mother's house. They came in and helped me clean out forty-nine years of my mother's accumulated stuff. They would pull everything out of the closets, drawers, and cabinets and then lay it all out so I could sort through it. I sorted by what to keep, donate, and trash. There was no time for a yard sale in my busy life. I also struck a bargain with the cleaning girls. I offered the cast-offs to them in lieu of money. It did save me several bucks and provided a bit of a laugh when their roller skate of a car left several times packed to where they could hardly close the car doors.

The plan was coming together bit by bit. The house took a few weeks to empty of memorabilia and junk, which included enough sheets to outfit the Klu Klux Klan and enough pots, pans, dishes, and silverware to feed them. Most of the wooden furniture was purchased by a local used furniture store. The soft furniture mostly went to whoever stopped by the side of the road on trash day. The sofas and chairs were from the early '60s and '70s and had seen better days.

I know at least some of the merchandise found a new home, since my office windows overlooked my mother's driveway, where the trash was piled. Each day, the scavengers would pick through the day's goodies. I don't know how much ended up in yard sales, basements, or college dorm rooms. It wasn't my merchandise, and my mother, even if she could remember each piece, did not need all that crap. She certainly did not need the six lawn and leaf bags full of Styrofoam packing peanuts, since she had not mailed a package to anybody in years. We did save several pieces of her stuff but already had enough of the right furniture to furnish her part of the house without overcrowding the space.

The plan started having problems even before the house was empty. I was not able to spend as much time in my mother's house because Lynne needed me more at my house. Plus I still had to set aside a few hours every day to visit my mother at Happy Valley.

Lynne did come with me on occasion to help clean or move things out of the house, but it was difficult to bring her along because of the stairs. The main reason I was consolidating into our house was, with Lynne's vision problems and the stairs into and inside my mother's house, it would be much more difficult for Lynne to navigate safely.

Then, of course, there was the little problem with the real estate bubble bursting. People in this neighborhood could not give their houses away. My neighborhood has historically been very popular, and it rarely took long to sell a house, no matter how bad the market had been. But I was in a position where I could wait for the market to improve, even though we were paying premium prices for my mother's little vacation at Happy Valley.

The biggest obstacle to overcome was cleaning the house to make it ready for the sale. The house was forty-nine years old, and my mother had lived in the house all forty-nine years. Don't get me wrong; she was not a packrat, hoarder, or slob. She just believed in saving a few things that may have some use one day. She also figured dusting and vacuuming was sufficient cleaning. Her curtains or blinds were usually closed, so she never realized that the windows could use a bit of sprucing up too.

Once the house was empty, I did a slow walk-through and made a list of what I needed to repair, replace, or clean and odds and ends that I might have to do after the initial sales push and feedback from potential buyers. Even though the house was nearly fifty years old, for the most part, it was in very good condition. But it did need a little paint inside and out, a bit of electrical updating, and a bathroom sink replacement—all in a day's work for me and what the checkbook could afford from the local pros.

Then came the serious cleaning of the hardwood floors that had never been more than dusted or swept. Three 1958-sized bedroom floors that needed to be cleaned by hand because every product the experts recommended would not cut the dirt enough to make it worth the time, effort, and money. I was on my hands and knees for an average of four hours nearly every day for over three weeks, board by board, getting nearly a half century of dirt off these floors. But when they were done, except for a few gouge marks, they shined like new. She would have been proud and probably a little embarrassed. I was sore but proud of how they turned out.

After the weeks of hands-and-knees cleaning of the floors, I turned my attention to cleaning the neglected windows. After having to replace the screens in ten of the fifteen windows, cleaning them was going to be a piece of cake, since they were tilt-in replacement windows. But nothing's easy in this life, especially when cleaning up someone else's mess. It seems that my mother, a sucker for every shyster handyman who came to the door, had a "brick preservative" sprayed on the house to extend the life of the bricks. When spraying this magic elixir, the contractor did not cover the windows, so each and every window pane was covered with a fine mist of some type of plastic. Needless to say, another task that should have taken a few hours ended up taking nearly two weeks.

What was the bottom line on getting my mother out of the house and getting it sold so we could move on with the modifications on my house? She moved into Happy Valley on October 15, 2007, and I sat in my living room, signing the settlement papers on April 30, 2010. Unfortunately, she passed on May 5, 2010. Even though she had no knowledge of the fix-up efforts, her eventual return to the neighborhood, or memory of the house, I guess somewhere deep inside she knew that she had nothing left to go back to.

So what's the moral of this story? Actually, there are two. Don't put off until tomorrow, and the best-laid plans. While my plan did not work out the way I planned, I know in my heart that while my mother vehemently disagreed, she was much better off at Happy Valley than in her house alone most of the time. Even though I was just a telephone call and less than two hundred feet away, I could not be in two places at the same time, and it was just a matter of time before she fell down the steps again, wandered away, or burned the house down.

Looking back on the whole escapade, I figured out where the flaws in my plan were. I underestimated how much work was required, and I did not factor in the number of times I went back and forth, responding to Lynne's needs. Something I also could not factor in was one of the snowiest winters on record, including three major snow storms within days of each other. I couldn't work on her house because I couldn't get to it.

Somewhere in the midst of cleaning out her house to prepare for the sale, it dawned on me that my mother had been showing signs of Alzheimer's disease in her shopping habits. When emptying the various closets and cabinets, we came across a treasure trove of cleaning products. I estimated that I would not have to buy laundry detergent, dish soap, and disinfectant cleaners for at least five years, since she had stockpiled these products, having forgotten that she had more than an ample supply from her previous trips to the store.

When cleaning out years of "collectibles," make sure to look everywhere. Look in everything, since people like to hide "valuables" inside boxes, books, cookie jars, and any number of unimaginable places. My mother was not such a hider that I was surprised when opening all of her pocketbooks and shoeboxes. I have heard of many families who have stumbled across hundreds or thousands of dollars, stock certificates, and insurance policies stuck inside books (especially the Bible). A former coworker discovered many stock certificates in his parents' attic that had been purchased in the infancy of a company named IBM and various other companies. Most had not fared as well as IBM as the years passed, but the fact remained there was a large sum of money that the family was not aware of.

The valuables that I uncovered or rediscovered were not of great monetary value, but the sentimental value was tremendous. The personal items that my mother had stored away in any number of dresser drawers included a well-worn Bible that her father had received from his mother in 1911 and another well-worn Bible that was given to my mother by her mother in 1933. I also unearthed a pocket-sized Bible that my father carried while he was in the Marine Corps.

The other sentimental treasures included the pocket watch that my great-grandfather and grandfather carried. I also located a well-worn 1890 silver dollar that was given to my grandfather by his grandfather. My grandfather carried this silver dollar in his pocket before, during, and after the Depression until he went to the hospital suffering from prostate cancer. But I found no vast sums of money, unknown insurance policies, or any other high-dollar treasures. I did find a stock certificate for a few shares of a long-defunct company based in Tennessee.

Use caution when cleaning out workshops, sheds, or barns following the demise of your loved one or when their cognitive skill set no longer allows them to work independently. A neighbor of ours, Jack, passed away a few years ago. He had spent his entire adult life in the construction field as a carpenter. After he passed away, his family cleaned out his tool shed and barn.

Many years ago, Jack brought home a small bottle containing a liquid to clean the chrome on his son's bicycle. He stored the remainder in his tool shed. This stored liquid had been in the tool shed for more than sixty years. Anna Lee, one of Jack daughter's, found this bottle and asked her brother what it was. It turns out this bottle contained nitroglycerin, which apparently could be used to clean chrome.

When Shirley, another of Jack's daughters, called the fire department to find out what to do with this antique nitroglycerin, the fire department responded that Shirley should set it down, and they would be right over. Within fifteen minutes, we had countless fire trucks and police cars from multiple jurisdictions determining what to do with this little bottle of well-aged nitroglycerin. Eventually, a representative from a military bomb squad arrived to assist in what to do and how to do it. We even had coverage by one of the local television stations.

To summarize the three-hour visit from the authorities, the fire department dug a hole away from all the houses and used the bomb squad robot to lift the bottle and carefully place the bottle in the hole. They were so unsure of the volatility and the potential destruction from this antique explosive that the neighbors were all evacuated from their homes. When the detonation occurred, it was little more than a thud and some flying dirt.

The bottom line is that cleaning out or cleaning up after a person's life can be interesting, revealing, or potentially dangerous. Be watchful and mindful, and above all else, have an escape route planned.

Caregiver's Shopping and Wish List

Any good professional in any field will tell you that you need the right equipment in order to do any job effectively and efficiently. Caregiving, like most professions, has its equipment and supplies. So that you are not overwhelmed by the caregiving items that you likely will need along the way, here is a quick shopping list of items, most of which I have found useful in caring for my mother and Lynne. Be mindful that if your victim enters hospice, necessary supplies and equipment are often paid for by Medicare, Medicaid, or private insurance. Also be mindful that your need for supplies and equipment will often occur before hospice will be in the picture to pick up the tab.

Some of these items may seem silly on the surface, may not apply to your particular situation, or may be too extravagant for your wallet. Check with your local churches and fraternal organizations before buying, since some have caregiving items that you can borrow. Also keep these groups in mind for the items that you purchased once you no longer need them.

Early preparation is a key component to keeping the scrambling to a minimum. Early preparation, such as buying supplies and equipment, also keeps the costs under control by allowing you to research the things you need or think you will need, comparison shop, and wait for sale prices. And if you do your buying online, you can wait for the free shipping offers.

- *Bed monitor.* Of all the tools I have amassed while caring for Lynne, the bed monitor is clearly the most useful piece of equipment in my caregiver's toolbox. It is particularly useful if your person is prone to getting out of bed or just sitting up in bed in the middle the night. I started using the monitor when Lynne would sit up in bed in the middle of the night. It warned me that she was uncovered and would get cold or could go back to sleep and fall out of bed. There are a variety of bed monitors to choose from. The basic types are a vinyl-covered pad that activates the alarm when the pressure is released, a pad that activates when pressure is applied, a physical connection using a clip on the clothing, and infrared beams. The type we use has a pad that activates a bedside alarm/transmitter, which sends a signal to the multilingual pager when pressure is released. I was told by a hospice nurse that the variety of bed alarm that hospice uses does not have this pager option, so the alarm is close to the bed and has been known to scare the patients. My best advice is to search the web and make some calls to make sure you get the type of monitor that fits your situation and budget.
- *Shower assist devices.* There are dozens of types of shower chairs, stools, or benches, but the principle is pretty much the same. The device sits either fully in the tub or half in and half out. The device that sits halfway out of the tub allows for the patient to sit on one end and slide across the bench into the tub without having to worry about any balance issues. The type we use, since Lynne's muscle control is poor at best, is a chair that swivels and slides on a track so she can sit down and I can position her in the tub without her having to do anything but sit and enjoy the ride. I will warn you that this half-in/half-out concept does not allow for the shower curtain to be fully closed, so expect water on the floor.

- *Handheld shower heads/shower wands.* Handheld shower devices make showering so much easier. They put the water where you need it. They vary widely in price and number of functions and are usually fairly easy to install.
- *Toilet seat elevator.* If your victim has sitting or standing issues, a toilet seat elevator will add a few inches to the height of the toilet seat.
- *Safety rails and grab bars in the bathroom.* You may want to enlist the assistance of a handyman or someone good with tools for this one. Safety rails and grab bars do not work well if not installed correctly.
- *Wheelchair.* I started using a wheelchair when Lynne's normal gait became more of a shuffle than a walk. This was supplied to me by hospice, so I had no out-of-pocket expense. Check the wheelchair suppliers for the wide variety of chairs and options if you need the chair before hospice comes in. As with the bed monitor, check the web and make a few calls. You would be amazed how many different wheelchairs there are and the wide range of prices and options.
- *Chair rail along the hallways.* This can help with maintaining balance as your loved one navigates the house. It can be very unobtrusive, is inexpensive, and can be removed once it is no longer needed.
- *Baby monitor.* A baby monitor that can be positioned by the bed or chair can cut down on your running back and forth, peeking around corners, and shouting through the house. It frees you to be in other parts of the house or out in the yard, depending on the range. I used a baby monitor with Lynne while I was working on readying my mother's house. The distance between the transmitter and receiver was roughly 175 feet. The signal was not crystal-clear, but I could hear anything that was being said on the television or radio, and I could hear Lynne, while she could still speak, if she needed anything. This

particular unit was not high-end. It was just a regular monitor bought off the shelf at a local department store.

- *Bed rails.* Obviously, the idea is to keep your AD victim in bed, and bed rails usually accomplish this. I, of course, have to use them differently. With the bed monitor and Lynne hardly moving while she is in bed, rails have not been necessary. But Lynne likes to sit on the corner of the bed, and as the disease progresses, she has developed what I call "target acquisition irregularities." Since she, like the rest of us, has no eyes on her butt (except mine), she would misjudge her target and end up sitting half on and half off the target. I use a bed rail across the bottom of the bed to give her a reference point, since she would bump into the bed rail before committing to the seated position, thus eliminating the fall risk.

- *Motion-activated lights and nightlights.* These can come in quite handy if your victim likes to roam around at night. These lights can cut down on tripping over or bumping into things. They also come in handy when you are navigating in the dark without having to grab for a flashlight or have to turn on a light. I have a motion-activated nightlight in nearly every room in the house. In power outages, they go on automatically and can be used as rechargeable flashlights. (Model: LED-92M available from *www.datexx.com.*)

- *Walking, safety, or transfer belt.* This may be necessary if the AD victim is too big for the caregiver to handle. There are several varieties to choose from. This belt, customarily a few inches wide, wraps around the patient's waist, allowing for better control by the caregiver. Some have handles built into the belt that make guiding and moving the patient easier. The number of handles depends on the size of the belt and the manufacturer.

- *Portable spot carpet cleaning machine.* Use this for cleaning up small accidents. A portable spot cleaning machine seems to be a luxury item until you have been on your hands and knees a few times. Accidents will happen whether they involve bodily fluids or solids, or spilled food or drink. These machines come in small sizes so that you are not overwhelmed or lose your closet space with a full-size unit. The smaller units are very convenient for tossing hot water and cleaning solution in and treating a spot on furniture or the floor.

- *Permanent or temporary ramps.* I cannot provide any personal information on this one since we live in a one-level house, and there is only one step at the front door to negotiate. If I were looking for a permanent ramp, I would talk to deck builders, handymen, or general contractors. For temporary or portable ramps I would turn to medical and wheelchair suppliers either locally or on the Internet.

- *Stand-alone generator.* These are quite pricey, and for some people, impractical or inconvenient. But I speak from experience, as we all do—when the lights go out because of a storm, you never know how many hours or days you will be in the dark. I determined, after thinking about it for a number of years, that we finally needed to buy a generator during a fifty-six-hour blackout after a summer thunderstorm knocked down most every power line in our area. We were fortunate that it was in the early part of the summer, so the temperature was not a big issue, and cooking was accomplished on the gas grill. But we did have to throw out everything in the refrigerator and freezer. The only time we have had to use the generator was following a snow and ice storm that put us in the dark on and off for five days. I fired up the generator after we had been in the dark for a few hours, and it was obvious from what I heard on the radio that we were in for a long-duration outage. With the generator running, we were able to keep the refrigerator and freezer cold, use the microwave, and have most of the lights, television, computer, and cell phone charger operational while everyone around us was in the dark. More importantly, we were able to keep our pellet stove running, keep the electric blanket on the bed warm and toasty, and operate the small space heater in the bathroom when it was needed. It was well worth the expense, and I would buy it again in a heartbeat. It's what I call cheap insurance. If you opt for a generator, remember three things. Do not use a generator in an unventilated area; make sure it is secured to something, since generators have been known to grow legs and walk away the longer the power is out and do a test run on occasions; and know that they can be quite noisy, so expect your jealous neighbors to offer up a few complaints.

- *Portable or window air conditioner and space heater.* Portable generators seldom have the power to run a whole-house HVAC system.

A few things you may already have at your disposal that on the surface sound like everyday conveniences may eventually become indispensable.

- *Microwave oven.* Cooking in a microwave beats slaving over a hot stove and cuts down on cooking time and cleanup to a certain degree.
- *Stick or immersion blender.* This is great for mixing smoothies and the like.
- *Slow cooker.* This cuts down on your time in the kitchen. It is great for making the type of meals that will become a staple as the disease progresses—stews and casseroles. Plus, you can stock up the freezer with these dishes.
- *Food processor.* This will become your best friend when your AD victim starts having issues with chewing and swallowing, and you don't want to feed him or her baby food.

If you have not been overwhelmed so far, add to your list home safety products like baby gates, which are especially important if you have a wanderer and stairs in your house. Anti-wandering devices can include door and window alarms, cow or jingle bells on doorknobs, and my personal favorite, which I use every day—a toothpick stuck into the casing around the door that offers enough resistance to prevent Lynne from opening the door easily if she turns the doorknob. But in an emergency the toothpick will break away quite easily with just a little more pressure. There are multiple upsides to this homemade quick fix: it costs next to nothing, is easily replaced and does not pose a safety hazard on either side of the door.

You may also consider extra sheets, blankets, towels, wash cloths, and whatever bed clothing your loved one prefers. My personal preference for Lynne's sleepwear has been V-neck cotton T-shirts. They are inexpensive, easy to clean, and will not tear if you have to rescue your victim in a fall. The extra sheets, blankets, towels, and wash cloths will likely come in handy at some point.

Then there is the daily stuff, such as disposable exam gloves, wee-wee pads, adult diapers, pre-moistened wipes (my personal favorite is ReadyBath), paper towels, straws, hand sanitizer (for you and any visitors), and personal cleaning supplies.

You have to approach caregiving for an adult with dementia no differently than preparing to care for a child who can get into anything and everything. The key to being prepared is coming to the realization that your fully grown loved one will likely need to be tended to like a large child—possibly one with an attitude. Also realize that my shopping list was for my application in my home, addressing my wife's needs. You likely will find other necessities as you go further with your AD victim.

Caregiving in the
Real World of Alzheimer's

I know that to new arrivals and the casual observer, this caregiving gig really does not look like a full-time job. But trust me when I say this—it is about the toughest job you could ever not ask for. The hours are long, the pay stinks, the benefits are nonexistent, and no matter how well you do your job today, you will probably have to do it again tomorrow—only better. Eventually, the job of caregiving will come to an end, and you will probably be okay with that for a number of reasons.

Many do not understand the role of the AD caregiver. Alzheimer's caregiving is a process that has no definitive roadmap. No matter who has been there before, while many have advice, they do not have concrete answers. Every AD victim is different, as is every caregiver, and if you work it right, you will survive the war even though you have lost many battles along the way.

Caregiving is finding the strength to carry on through the sleepless nights and never-ending days while ignoring the exhaustion, boredom, and loneliness that must you face every day, whether you like it or not. Whether you are caregiving because of love, some misunderstood obligation, or the lack of money for assisted living, your goal is quite simple—to persevere.

At the adult level, caregiving relies more on instinct than anything that can be learned from a book, especially with diseases that attack the brain and chip away at every part of the victim's cognitive skill set the further the disease progresses, thus limiting what you have to work with. Alzheimer's caregiving is much the same as the caregiving involved in most any other disease. But what separates caregivers for the memory challenged from other caregivers? The memory challenged care recipients may not recognize their caregivers, usually do not remember why they need assistance, and may not remember who they themselves are.

Someone—usually a loved one—depends on others for food, hygiene, safety, and companionship. But every day, the struggles often revolve around not just the tasks at hand, but convincing the victim that it is okay for you to do your job and that he or she has nothing to be concerned about. The loss of memory, especially short-term memory, puts the caregiver at a distinct disadvantage every day. You often need to start from scratch, sometimes fighting the paranoia of being a stranger to your loved one, just to get the simplest of tasks accomplished.

Short-term memory loss does not allow for new skills to be taught or old skills to be reinforced, and sometimes it does not allow for a smooth transition for the caregiver to take over. Even though the care recipient has been doing these everyday tasks for decades, this does not mean you can remind them or expect them to remember no matter how many times you encourage them to remember.

Imagine being in a strange house with a person you do not know who wants to give you pills you do not remember ever having taken before or know the reason for. How about the same stranger putting his or her hands on you—especially your private parts? (I know some people pay big bucks for this, but that's off the point.) Put yourself in the victim's shoes when the questions you ask the stranger are answered with words like, "Trust me."

My father's illness and death put me in the position of having to be the "man of the house" at age twelve. It also gave me some perspective on how to deal with the problems that come with caring for someone with a terminal disease.

I am the sole caregiver for my wife, who, at the time of this writing, is in the late stages of Early Onset Alzheimer's disease. While I have no formal training as a caregiver, I think (and many professional and nonprofessional caregivers agree) that I do an excellent job of meeting all of Lynne's needs. At the end of the day, she has been fed, clothed, bathed, medicated, watched by loving eyes, guided by dedicated hands, and kept as safe as humanly possible. In short, she's not left wandering down the road, left hungry, or left alone for more than a moment on a typical day. And in the Alzheimer's game, most days are anything but typical—but we somehow manage to weather the storm every day. For those who think I need help to care for my best friend in her daily struggle, I beg to differ. I am not so stubborn or prideful not to ask for help before I get in over my head. After all, caregiving is determining what is best for the person being cared for and certainly not about the caregiver and the caregiver's ego.

My outlook on this slow-motion train wreck is quite simple. Anticipate and prepare for all of the worst-case scenarios, and be happy when I have been overly concerned, or God forbid, overly prepared. I am here to tell you that the logistics of caregiving are drastically different from victim to victim and caregiver to caregiver. I know this firsthand, having cared for two Alzheimer's victims simultaneously and having observed numerous dementia patients while visiting my mother at Happy Valley nearly every day for over two years. This gave me the opportunity to study actions of other dementia victims and the responses of their professional caregivers as well as how family members interacted with their demented loved ones.

The quality of care I provide for my wife is just plain obvious, even to passing strangers. She is clearly sick, fragile, confused, unsteady, and easily distracted. But more than that, she is and always will be my wife, my love, and my best friend. To say I would do anything for her is an understatement. Many have seen and understand this without me saying a word. I will talk to anybody who will listen about our situation in hope that they will see and understand not just the level of commitment I have for her care but also the love. While, on the surface, it may sound like I'm bragging, I am really not. It is not my way. I expect no pat on the back, no caregiver of the year award, or any sympathy for my role in Lynne's life as it comes to a premature end.

When Lynne was diagnosed, it was solely up to me to determine what was available for helping her and what (if anything) was available for helping me support her increasing needs. Even though I already had some knowledge of the disease following my mother's diagnosis, I knew, based on their different symptoms, I needed more information. I researched the disease, and on the recommendation of Lynne's neurologist, found various clinical trials and pursued them—again, with very little help.

Simple requests like asking for Lynne's very brief file to be faxed by the neurologist's office to the clinical trial coordinator at Georgetown apparently fell on deaf ears (twice). At the time, I was dealing with the neurologist's less-than-motivated front office staff, the Georgetown clinical trial coordinator, and caring for my mother and my wife, so I certainly did not need the "assistance" of yet another paper-pushing front office staffer. My job was to ask nicely, expect useless assistance, and get Lynne into a clinical trial.

While every symptom seems to be worse for Lynne than most everyone else, and my mother was a textbook example of symptoms, I had to keep both in mind when making decisions. When my mother was solely my responsibility, I had to make decisions regarding her care while considering how it would impact Lynne. It was often a balancing act, since my mother rarely recognized that she needed assistance and would quite often reject anything I would say or do that would encroach on her independence. So did I have to work harder to care for both of them simultaneously? I did not necessarily have to work harder, but I certainly had to work smarter, since I would have to analyze the entire situation from both sides before making changes, no matter who was affected directly.

I know I am carrying a heavy burden, caring for Lynne single-handedly. I know that people want what is best for both of us, and I certainly do understand and appreciate their concern. Several times, I have been offered assistance in the form of CNAs and volunteers through hospice. But I know the pieces of the Lynne care puzzle better than anyone who could walk into the house to care for her for a few hours when I need a break. I almost always know what she wants or needs, even though her needs are constantly changing. I know her patterns, facial expressions, and body language. And why do I get a break from my responsibilities when Lynne doesn't get a break from her disease? I will take my break when Lynne no longer needs my assistance. While I certainly do appreciate the offer from hospice for respite care, I see the future, and if I accept the offer of assistance, once they are out the door, I still have to pick up the pieces, which means more work for me.

I did at one time avail myself of an offer of assistance from a hospice CNA (Certified Nursing Assistant), who would help Lynne get a shower. It was really an experiment to determine Lynne's acceptance of a stranger and my willingness to briefly relinquish control. I know Lynne was uncomfortable with the situation. She did not really understand who this new person was, but after a few minutes of my reassurance, she did except the offer of assistance from this stranger.

The CNA did an acceptable job of assisting Lynne, but the aftermath left me with two hours of detangling Lynne's waist-length hair. I am not sure if the few minutes of the shower assistance and my respite was worth the two hours of the detangling. But what I do know is that was the last shower assistance I received and the last assistance I requested. I have too much to do to have to undo someone else's handiwork while putting Lynne through the discomfort of the unknown person and the bigger discomfort of me having to detangle her long hair. But like I have often said, hopefully you learn from your mistakes and move on.

When you first start taking care of your loved one, your normal life becomes a list of minor modifications in your lifestyle while accommodating their changes in attitude or cognitive skills. As the disease progresses, your job becomes one of figuring out what your loved one needs or when they need it—sometimes with little information to go on other than a frown, grunt, some disjointed chatter, or a rant based on something you have done that does not meet with expectations. Or their needs may have nothing to do with you at all. And as attuned to your loved one's needs as you are, it is easy to become complacent because you are so close to the situation and usually see the changes as they occur without realizing it. But you may overlook new changes or make a mistake, hurt feelings, or just not understand what is required of you. Welcome to the world of Alzheimer's caregiving!

Caregiving is part art, part science, part guesswork, and part prayer. It is a process of learning as you go while being as flexible as humanly possible, recognizing that you are human and can make mistakes while finding out what works today in the situation that you are currently facing. At many points, you may have to change your regular way of doing things, even though you have been doing these things the same way for months or even years, because your victim has decided that you are not doing it the right way. Usually you discover this in a standoff, quite often out of the clear blue sky. This is where you can score big points by staying ahead of the changes, even though you do not know what the changes will be. You can think quickly on your feet to develop a plan B when the changes occur. No matter how trivial the changes are, they have to be addressed when they happen. What separates the successful caregiver from the also-rans is seeing and responding to changes with little disruption in care while not taking anything said or done by the victim personally.

I am not complaining any more than any other person watching a loved one slowly being destroyed by disease. But when Lynne got the Alzheimer's list of symptoms, she got them all, and she has shown every one of them throughout the disease. As she continues to decline, no matter what I do to compensate, my actions will often be effective for only a short period of time. That is what makes AD caregiving quite a challenge. It's not just about the anticipated increase in existing symptoms, but also about new symptoms that present themselves through the progression of the disease. It's like somebody changed the rules of the game in the middle of the game, and you didn't get a copy of the new rules.

Alzheimer's caregiving goes in stages. Unfortunately, as you develop a routine, you will find out that the disease, the care recipient, or both will decide it is time to move on to the next stage. No matter how well you fulfill your caregiving duties the victim and the disease ultimately will decide what you have to do and when you have to do it. The AD victim and the disease call the shots, and there is rarely negotiation or advanced warning.

Even though needs will increase and timing will change, you should try to develop a schedule—albeit an extremely flexible one that is always subject to change—so caregiving and other responsibilities can be managed. For several years, nearly every night, I would answer the bed alarm roughly one hour after Lynne went to bed. Then the alarm would go off again one hour later. The third time the bed alarm would go off as much was two hours later. So it was possible to develop a schedule around Lynne's sleep pattern, because it was very consistent for a few years. That's not to say that we did not have nights when she did not go to bed until after eleven o'clock, which tended to throw the entire time chart out the window. And there were a few nights in years ten through twelve when she has actually slept through the night. One night, in year eleven, she went to bed unusually early after a particularly trying day. She slept through the first potty run. Then the second went by. About three hours after she went to bed, I actually checked to make sure she was still breathing. Between her near-motionless sleep and her very dependable sleep schedule, I was quite concerned.

Here is a quick list of things to do as you dive headfirst into the craft of caregiving. It may be harsh to say, but you really have to prepare the home as if you are caring for small children who can and will get into anything and everything the moment your back is turned. Start by packing, hiding, or locking up things that could become safety issues—knives, razors, scissors, tools, guns, medicines (prescription and over-the-counter), poisons, and breakables. Remember, if you found a hiding place, chances are your loved one will too. This list of changes and preparations will get longer when you start seriously looking around your house inside and out. Do not overlook barns, sheds, off-site storage units, the car, RV, or boat. Why make a bad situation even worse by spending time in the emergency room (or worse) because of something that should have been stored, tossed, or disabled?

If you have planned to paint or redecorate, do it sooner rather than later so your victim will at least have some chance of getting used to the new paint or new furniture, and you still have the time to get the work done.

At some point in time, you will realize that you have become the parent of your grandparent, parent, or spouse. Or you may have to reestablish your position as parent to your grown child. This is the part of caregiving that, if you haven't had too many problems, can begin to erode the relationship the two of you have had, no matter how strong it was before dementia entered the picture. The victim will likely fight you at every opportunity because he or she knows you are not helping. You are holding them hostage and treating him or her like a child.

"Will I get better?" "Why am I this way?" "Why do I take these pills?" or questions to that effect will be coming at some point in time. Diminished thought process or not; your loved one will ask questions. You better have an answer, and "because" is just not going to cut it. No matter how incapacitated AD victims are and will become, they are still thinking, functioning adults who deserve more than just food and clean clothes. They deserve your respect, no matter how many unusual requests or demands they make on you. If you don't respect them and respect what they are going through while fighting this life-ending disease, then you missed the whole point of being a caregiver. They are going to ask questions, usually when you least expect it. You should be prepared with a satisfying answer to their questions without delay or deflection.

So with all this being said about understanding, caring, and respecting, what do you do with questions and objections that arise to which you don't have the answer your loved one wants to hear? A well-crafted lie or creative story never hurt anyone, especially if it keeps the victim content, keeps the medications or food onboard, and keeps you from having to sing and dance your way out of the corner.

After my mother moved to Happy Valley, she would frequently refuse to take her medications. The answer was simple—a little creative storytelling. I would tell her the doctor would not let her go home until she took her medicine. Another favorite was that the medicine was for her diabetes, and if she didn't take the pills, she could end up like her cousin, who lost both legs to diabetic neuropathy.

My mother resisted the Happy Valley staff almost constantly, even though she had been around most of them for as much is two years. So if you meet resistance because "I don't know who you are," don't feel like you have done something wrong. This is the disease making sure it gets in the way as much as possible. And like I said before, you cannot be too prepared. This "who are you" problem normally comes out of the blue. Prepare to be blindsided because you are not who you say you are; you are whoever the AD victim thinks you said you are.

As if we don't have enough to worry about and our victims don't have enough problems, we have the ever-present possibility of agitation, combativeness, or loss of inhibition—all breakdowns of a personality that the pre-Alzheimer's victim developed over a lifetime. The disease is destroying what made the person who he or she used to be. And for better or worse, the disease is determining who he or she will become.

One of the problems some AD victims experience is the loss of inhibition. It is the control mechanism inside our heads that controls how we generally act around other people. It keeps most of us from blurting out profanity, making racial comments, and taking off our pants in public. Agitation or combativeness can often become an issue when caring for AD victims. The confusion or inability to do what they know they can do often leads to lashing out at the closest target. Usually it is you, since you are the closest person, and in your loved one's mind, you are most likely responsible for their loss. You will always be in your AD victim's crosshairs.

Keep in mind that even though you have "dementia-proofed" the house by removing any possible weapons that an AD victim could lay hands on, do not forget they can still use their hands and probably will not hesitate to use them if prompted by you overstepping your bounds, even though you are the person trying to help. No matter how much you may be tempted, you cannot handcuff or tie your loved one up. Not only is this dangerous, illegal, and potentially kinky, but it is also just not fair.

But before you give up hope of controlling an overly agitated AD victim, talk with the doctors about the situation—preferably before it gets out of control. Most likely, they will send you out to the pharmacy for a little brown bottle of "instant answers." I am not a big proponent of brown-bottle therapy, but sometimes you have to do what you have to do. But before you take the instant answers approach, try to take a step back, honestly reexamine your caregiving techniques, and if possible, determine what set off your loved one. The first question I asked myself when my mother became more verbally demanding and frequently agitated should be the same question you ask yourself: "Am I trying to control her too much?" I've been there, done that, and learned from it.

Time becomes a near-useless commodity as the disease progresses and your workload increases. The regimented lifestyle that we all lived under before Alzheimer's—up in time for work, eat meals at a set time, watch television at certain times, and go to bed at a regular time—is old business because you have now entered "the caregiver time zone." (Cue *The Twilight Zone* theme music.) With the exception of doctor's appointments, medication schedules, and the like, you can just toss the time schedule and the clock. Your loved one and the disease usually decide what time to do most everything.

It makes my skin crawl when someone tells me to have a good weekend. Who has a weekend? I stopped having days of the week after my mother moved into Happy Valley. Gone by the wayside were weekdays and weekends because every day—no matter what the calendar says—is today, and your loved one likely does not know or remember what day, date, or season it is anyway. I did at one time have yesterday, today, and tomorrow. Yesterday was for the things I said I did or should have done. Tomorrow was for the things I wanted to avoid doing or talking about. Today is the only time that is real, and you can't hide from it. I did occasionally have last week or next month for my mother's questions or concerns that I wanted to avoid talking about entirely.

—————ༀ∘ᄋᄂᄋᄁᄋᄀᄋ∘ᄋᄱ—————

Quite often, the responsibilities of performing the ADLs plus your non-caregiving responsibilities will overshadow the quiet times you will want or need to have with your loved one. Some caregivers will play cards or games, read, do various craft projects, go for walks, or just sit and talk about the old days while leafing through scrapbooks or photo albums with their AD victims.

Beginning in the middle stages of Lynne's affliction, I read the balance of the Harry Potter book she had started. Then I read stories from magazines and newspapers that she would have enjoyed before the AD stole her ability to read. And I read to her from the Mormon Bible, which she found enjoyable because I would do various accents and sound effects during my reading. But the number one thing I did—and still do—to help us remain somewhat normal is to make it my daily mission to try to make her smile or laugh at least one time. That is what makes us normal. I strongly suggest that if you have the time and are not doing any of the above or activities similar to them, give them a try because they may give you or your loved one a little peace of mind. It is also a way for you to sit and relax while still in caregiving mode.

———————

It is important that you keep notes on your victim's condition and your caregiving efforts. These notes will come in handy should you decide to pursue clinical trials, if you need to change doctors, apply for Social Security Disability benefits, apply for state or local programs for assistance, and believe it or not, defend your actions to family members who think they could do a better job but are not willing to step up to the plate. This disease, like any other terminal disease, can and will bring out the best or worst in everybody—no matter what role they play. So don't get caught with your pants down. Keep your notes just in case because you never know when they will come in handy. If you start making notes early on, you will become accustomed to doing it, and you won't be scrambling around at the last minute, trying to figure out what happened, when it happened, and where it happened. The best use I found for keeping records and notes is that since you will probably lose your mind doing this caregiving thing, you can look back at the various disasters and say, "Ah, the good old days."

A neighbor of ours received a not-so-courteous visit from the authorities when someone called the county elder care office regarding the care her father was receiving. Again, someone was butting in with no direct knowledge of the situation. She had to defend herself to the authorities after they essentially raided her father's home. Fortunately, she had been doing her best, and they found no elder abuse violations. Keep notes on your caregiving efforts in case you have a busybody neighbor or relative who wants to ride in and save the day.

———∿∿⦿⦿⦿∿———

Weight loss and loss of appetite often will come along during the course of the disease. Before you spend hours in the kitchen fixing your AD victim's favorite foods, remember that one of the early and often-overlooked symptoms of Alzheimer's disease is the loss of sense of smell. And with a change or loss of sense of smell, food can take on a different taste.

When Lynne's appetite started falling off, I went through the recipe books, trying to find foods that might entice her taste buds. Her previous favorites had no more reaction than dry toast or a glass of water. So I went to the opposite direction to prove a point. Lynne has always hated peanut butter. If Mary and I did not make PB&J for the kids when they were growing up, they would have never had it, since Lynne so hated peanut butter. I fed Lynne peanut butter on a few occasions, and she had no reaction. That told me her sense of smell was certainly out of order, and trying to entice her to eat even her favorites was foolhardy at best.

———∿∿⦿⦿⦿∿———

There will come a time when asking questions of your cognitively challenged loved one will become more trial and error than a simple request for information. When asking questions of your AD loved one, keep a few things in mind to hopefully limit confusion or misunderstandings.

- Avoid lengthy, multiple-choice questions.
- Avoid inferences or reading between the lines.
- Keep your questions short and to the point. Too much information in your question just makes your AD victim remember more than their mind is likely capable of digesting.

- Don't expect an instant answer. Give your AD victim a chance to answer one question at a time or allow them to answer your question with more questions.
- Limit your use of pronouns, and make sure your nouns and pronouns agree.

A simple question of personal comfort may seem straightforward enough. Your typical question of comfort to your loved one may sound like this: "Are you hot, cold, or comfortable, and do you need help taking off your sweater?" But with the limited thought process available, as little as three options becomes a laundry list to someone with a cognitive deficit. This just makes the already confused mind have to work harder, which simply frustrates the victim—and eventually, you. What in our minds (and formerly the minds of AD victims) seems to be a no-brainer (sorry) in fact becomes several pieces of an already jumbled puzzle.

Failure in caregiving comes not only from poor planning, but also from forgetting that no matter how diligent or well-prepared you are, the disease itself will change or challenge your well-laid plans without warning. Contrary to what you may believe or hope, your Alzheimer's victim is unable to keep cognitive changes from occurring. But your cognitively challenged loved one may be able to play you like a fiddle once they see your reactions. Somehow AD victims always remember that part. It becomes a fine line between what the Alzheimer's has done and how your AD victim interprets your reactions. Remember, your loved one is sick, not stupid.

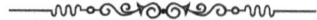

There is a problem with short-term memory loss and ADLs. You just spent thirty minutes feeding your loved one. You are sitting at the table, and the dirty dishes are still sitting there. Then what happens? "I'm hungry; when do we eat?" In your even, calm voice, you respond that you have just eaten, and you will be eating again in a few hours. If you don't get too much opposition, you will come away with a sense of accomplishment because you handled the situation very well. You said no cross words, did not avoid the situation, and above all, you won this small skirmish. Unfortunately, your cognitively challenged loved one does not remember the food. They just remember that you are starving them and refusing to feed them.

———⁓⁓⋯⊙⋯⊙⋯⁓⁓———

It is absolutely necessary to have your emergency contact information up-to-date. Carry it with you whenever you leave the house, and have it posted in an obvious place in your house. It is what I keep saying and can never say enough—be prepared for the most unlikely situation, such as being in a car accident on that ten-minute run to the drugstore while your loved one is sitting at home unattended.

This emergency contact information consists of more than just whom to call if something happens. Even though there is very little timetable in an Alzheimer's house, your emergency contact information should indicate anything on a schedule, such as medication and feeding times. Also make note of any unusual comfort items your AD victim may need, like a special blanket, stuffed animal, or item of clothing. The long and the short of it is that you need to have documentation so whoever comes in to take over for you, whether temporary or permanent, knows at least the basics of the care plan and can implement it without the same learning process that you went through. This hopefully will ensure that your loved one will have a continuity of care.

Whenever the potential for dangerous weather exists, you should dress your victim and have an emergency bag with medications, caregiving instructions, cash, and emergency contact information packed. You don't want to be dressing your AD victim and grabbing essentials as a storm is bearing down on you. Try to show your loved one that you are concerned but not panicking about a possible emergency if he or she realizes you are doing something unusual.

A medic alert necklace or bracelet with your victim's name, condition, address, and your cell phone number is an extremely important safety measure for the AD victim. You never know if you and your victim could become separated during a regular outing, in an emergency, or if he or she wanders. And we all know that Alzheimer's will usually get in the way of a successful reunion. Have recent photographs on your cell phone or other electronic device, or just have photographs with you when you and your AD victim are out in the real world. Also make a mental note of what your loved one is wearing every day.

———— ⁓⊶⊙⊷⊙⊶⊙⊶⊙⊷⊙⊶⊙⊶⁓ ————

Just when you are absolutely positive that you have seen it all, heard it all, done it all, and there's nothing new under the sun when it comes to caring for your loved one, AD will sneak up on you and throw you a curve. If you are lucky, an emergent problem or situation can be handled without too many additional problems. Hopefully, there will be no long-lasting residue that you have to clean up later (literally or figuratively).

After dinner one evening in year eleven, I left Lynne sitting on the love seat in the great room while I cleaned up the kitchen. I had been in the kitchen for about two or three minutes when I heard an unusual cough. So I decided to check on Lynne. I came into the room, and there stood Lynne with her back to me. I spoke as I approached so I would not frighten her. As I got closer, she turned slightly to show me what was happening.

There she stood, covered in blood from forehead to foot—big spots, little spots, and smears of fresh blood. She looked like the color version of an old gangster who was brought down in a hail of gunfire. She had somehow caused her nose to bleed—and bleed it did! The blood was pouring out—far more than any nosebleed I had ever seen. So with my high school first aid training and experience of more than a few nosebleeds of my own, I was able to quickly get the bleeding under control, though it did take me a while to clean up the residue. Nearly every exposed part of Lynne—her clothes, the cover on the love seat, the floor, and Genie—all had been bloodied. I cleaned blood into the night and the following morning. There's never a dull moment here in Realityville!

———

The Internet is full of "it worked for us" cure and treatment articles and videos touting the value of some bizarre foods, magic vitamin combinations, or some mystical herbs from the jungles of an unheard-of land. I am not saying that these treatments are bogus, but use your brain before "curing" your victim into uncontrollable vomiting and diarrhea, a coma, or an earlier grave. Talk with your victim's doctors to determine if there is any validity to these claims of a better treatment or cure and if there are any possible side effects or conflicts with the medications currently being used should you decide to attempt one of these website miracle cures.

One of the few "it worked for us" articles I came across addressed the use of aromatherapy—not as a cure or treatment, but as a way to calm and comfort. Sometimes familiar aromas can remind the cognitively challenged of people, past events, or once-familiar locations. The article listed different aromas and combinations of aromas that have certain effects on people who do not have cognitive impairments. I felt that this was not harmful or a potential conflict with medications, so I started experimenting with different aromas and gauged their effects on Lynne. I found that lavender was the most effective in helping her to be more alert. I found nothing that would act as a calming aroma, which was okay, since Lynne seldom needs calming. But I was also hoping to use this experiment on my mother to help her be less agitated. I never had the opportunity to try it out on my mother, so I cannot report on aromatherapy and its calming effects.

———————

If you leave your cognitively challenged loved one home alone, be aware of the obvious safety hazards, like fires, falls, and wandering. Also know the AD victim may let strangers in the house. Other than the obvious dangers to life and property, they might sign contracts with shyster home repairmen, give large sums of money to anyone who knocks on the door, or let the family pet out. They could also buy merchandise over the telephone or online. Let's face it—there's always something else to watch out for. Also remember your AD victim may have known you when you left a few hours ago, but there is no guarantee they will know you when you return.

"Ruth," a woman in the middle stages of Alzheimer's, was living alone and was apparently doing well with the part-time assistance of her sister, "Judy," who would stay with Ruth for about ten hours every day. When Judy got to the house every morning, she would announce herself so as to not scare Ruth. One morning, when Judy arrived, after announcing her presence, she was unable to find Ruth. Judy, fearing something had happened to her sister during the night, started looking everywhere. When Judy swung open a closet door, Ruth lunged at her with a knitting needle. Fortunately, the wound was relatively minor, requiring some stitches, a little gauze, and a tetanus shot.

I have seen and heard it over and over—planning or attending a special event involving an Alzheimer's victim. In my opinion, once an AD victim is having difficulties identifying close family members or remembering major past events with any level of clarity, having that special event or outing so they will "at least have the memory before they go" just sets you up for disappointment and the victim for more confusion, frustration, or possible danger. And if you deal with a wanderer or an exhibitionist, these special events are just opportunities for disaster. Also, other participants in this event will likely be focused on the event and not the victim. Let's face it; we're all human.

We are dealing with a disease where the most common symptom is short-term memory loss. Chances are excellent that the only memories of this special event will be yours, and they will be less than the magic moments you were hoping for. You most certainly will be disappointed when your Alzheimer's victim—the one who struggles to remember who you are—does not remember the next day that you had this special event or outing.

I am not saying to keep your loved one tied to the bed or a tree in the backyard, but just remember whom and what you are dealing with. This caregiving job is full of disappointments and setbacks in normal conditions. Do not add to your list of disappointments if you can possibly avoid it. Trust me when I say this—there are plenty of disappointments in store for you and your AD victim in just trying to live a normal life from day to day.

Even though your life is consumed with the care of your loved one, life is still going on in the world around you. You know it's going to happen at some point in the downward spiral of Alzheimer's. Some event will occur that you feel will cause so much turmoil in your AD victim's mind that you feel the need to protect them from it. These events can be the catastrophic type, like death or serious injury of someone close. Then again, in your mind, the event could be a minor concern. But in the AD victim's altered thought process, this minor situation may seem to be a major problem.

So you ask yourself, *What do I do?* In my mother's case, I was a very strong proponent of, "What she doesn't know can't hurt me." This certainly served me well on more than the rare occasion. You may think this is the chicken's way out, and you would be absolutely correct. But not telling the person has a way of coming back and biting you on the butt at the least opportune time because somehow the secret finds its way out into the open. No matter how many times you tell everyone, "Don't say anything about . . ." it always finds a way of slipping out because someone wasn't in the information loop, just forgot, or wants to be a know-it-all and spill the beans.

While my mother was at the rehabilitation facility recuperating from her broken hip, and several weeks after she returned home, she suffered the loss of a number of people in her life. During her down time, she lost a cousin whom she helped raise, a friend of the family who was like a son to my grandmother and like a brother to my mother, and at least two other people she was close to. But the biggest loss was the unexpected death of her nephew, Mark.

Mark was the older of my mother's sister's two children. He was a very special individual, and my mother thought the world of him. I knew his passing would be hard on her, since she was always very concerned about Mark—especially after her sister, Buddy, passed away.

Mark's death occurred while my mother was still at the rehabilitation facility. I got the call one Saturday morning from Mark's sister-in-law, Carla. She told me that Mark had passed away and wanted to know how we should handle telling my mother. This news was devastating, and the AD added an unknown element to how strongly she would react. Before the Alzheimer's, this news would have certainly been hard for her to handle.

We determined it was best for me to break the bad news, since I was with my mother in Virginia and Carla was in Iowa. I would be in the best position to determine when my mother was up to hearing the bad news and what words I should use to lessen the blow. Between the Alzheimer's and the various drugs being used for pain management and to keep her calm, I was initially unsure how and when to approach telling her about Mark's passing.

According to the rehabilitation schedule, I had roughly four weeks to figure out how and when I would tell her before she was scheduled to come home. Since she was not receiving telephone calls and had few visitors other than Lynne and me, there was no danger that someone would let it slip. The few other potential visitors would not be told until my mother was informed so I could pick my opportunity to break the bad news on my terms, keeping in mind her fragile state and the love she had for her deceased nephew.

To say my mother was not content at the rehab facility is, at best, an understatement. Much of the time, she was given medications to help her "relax." She was in a strange environment in a semiprivate room on a very busy hallway, so she had almost no privacy. I did not want to tell her of Mark's death in front of a crowd for two reasons. It was nobody's business except ours, and I was not sure how strongly my mother would react. I also felt it would be better to be at the rehab facility with the nurses a few feet away in case she had an extreme reaction.

My mother's roommate was bedridden but had frequent doctor's appointments that took her from the facility for several hours at a time. So I waited for my mother to have a good day while the roommate had one of her doctor days to break the news.

The opportunity to have this shoebox-sized, semiprivate room to ourselves finally arrived. Lynne and I had our customary visit, where we would put my mother in her wheelchair, go to the sunroom, sit and chat for a while, and then return to the room. On the way back to her room, I spoke with the charge nurse to determine if my mother's roommate had returned. I got the response I was hoping for; the roommate was still out and probably would be out for a few more hours. I informed the charge nurse that I had bad news to give my mother regarding a death in the family, and I had waited to tell her because of the privacy issues as well is my mother's overall condition. I told the nurse that I would be informing my mother of Mark's death in the next few minutes and that I may need some assistance, depending on how strong my mother's reaction was.

With all the pieces of the puzzle falling into place, I was ready to drop the bomb. After getting my mother out of the wheelchair and back into bed, I shut the door. I got my mother's attention and calmly told her that I had spoken with Carla and that she had some bad news about Mark. I told her that Mark had suffered a stroke and had passed away, that it was quick, and he did not suffer. The silence was deafening while she processed the news. A few moments of silence broke way to a flood of tears, but there was no major breakdown. She cried for a while, stopping every few minutes to ask what happened, when it happened, and the like. I think she was verifying what I had said rather than needing to have the details about what happened. About fifteen minutes after I broke the news, the charge nurse came to check on my mother and offer her condolences. She also had a syringe and a vial in her possession just in case my mother needed some assistance.

About an hour after my mother stopped crying and had calmed down, Lynne and I left. As we were leaving, we thanked the nurse for her visit and the kind words, which were somewhat unexpected, since my mother had run the nursing staff ragged for most of her stay. We returned a few hours later to make sure that my mother was okay and to sit with her if she wanted company. We arrived to find her smiling and talking with her roommate and an aide, telling stories about Mark. It was like she was giving his eulogy.

In the time after rehab and before going to Happy Valley, my mother would frequently call Mark's brother, David, to check on the family. Of course, the conversation would turn to how Mark was doing. Even though I told her numerous times of Mark's death, the short-term memory loss would not allow this new memory to take hold, which continued to put David and Carla in the awkward position of having to decide how to answer my mother's questions concerning Mark.

I could identify with their problem. Addressing the subject of dead family and friends was something I had been dealing with almost daily with my mother. As the disease continued to erase her memory, I was faced with having to break the bad news day after day—sometimes several times a day—of the loss of my grandparents, my father, and any number of friends and relatives. At that stage, I felt that honesty was the best policy, since she could just pick up the telephone and verify any information I gave her on most anybody. After she entered Happy Valley, I felt it was better to resurrect the dead and let her know that whomever she was asking about was still alive and well and that I had spoken with them recently. After all, she could not verify anything I said, as she had no access to the telephone, and with few exceptions, she had no visitors other than me.

Let's face it—all things being equal, at the end of the day, no matter how bad it has been today, tomorrow is a new day full of hope and promise for a better outcome than the day before. The one prayer or hope we all share is that tomorrow will be a better day and that we will have the strength to see it through, no matter what surprises we have in store. But know this—you will lose this war, no matter how hard you fight, no matter how passive or aggressive you are, and no matter how much help you receive. There is an end to this war. If you can look back once your job is done and feel that you did everything you could for your AD victim, more often than not, you have, in fact, won the war, and they are in a better place.

Nichole and I often say that we are both on the same road—just going in opposite directions. With every cognitive downturn Lynne suffers and I have to find a way to compensate, it seems that Nichole is going the opposite direction with our young grandson, Zechariah. As he is learning to talk, Lynne is losing her ability to speak, and I have to come up with ways to understand her needs. This is no different from Nichole needing to translate young Zechariah's words into actions. As Zechariah is learning all of the skills that will serve him through life, like walking, talking, using the bathroom, and learning about the great big world around him, Lynne is going in the exact opposite direction.

Does caregiving ever get any easier? The early stages require more of a wait-and-see approach while doing little things to cover your loved one's mistakes. The challenges are normally small and can be compensated for, and you spend most of your time saying, "Don't worry about it." The middle stages of AD can really be compared to the "terrible twos." Along with the good times, it seems that every day is filled with questions, pouting, rage, distrust, and the occasional potty accident.

Yes, personally, I think it gets slightly easier the further into the disease we go. But that's not to say that any of this nightmare is ever easy, and it is seldom routine. But as time goes on, a level of trust and dependency will hopefully develop. Hopefully, your AD victim recognizes you as their source for food, ADL, and companionship. They hopefully have developed trust in the stranger you have become who is doing the right thing for them. Your loved one's comfort with you as the caregiver should make it easier to get through each day. But the later stages are truly twenty-four hours a day—constantly putting out fires, patching boo-boos, cleaning up missteps, and not being able to relax for more than a moment at a time. But it is easier, since you have had, in most cases, years of preparation. You often know what to expect and have the tools and experience to fix most any problem when it arises. So does it ever any get easier? Yes. No. Maybe. Sometimes.

Controlling the
Caregiving Environment

After you have secured all the dangerous objects in the house, installed whatever safety and anti-wandering devices you may require, and procured the supplies you need, there is something you should seriously consider that may help keep your AD victim more comfortable and less restless. You may want or need to control the AD victim's environment, so it is more comfortable for them. These environmental elements could include lighting, temperature, furniture placement, colors or patterns on bedding or curtains, and the list could be nearly endless. It may take a while to figure out any glitches, so be patient, but be proactive. Trust me on this one—you will want to revisit the environmental part of the caregiving plan several times, as it may need adjustment as the seasons change and the victim becomes more cognitively challenged.

The bottom line is to find anything (within reason) that will help you help your AD victim. Generally, what is good for the care recipient should be good for you and your caregiving efforts. You may also be the missing answer to why your loved one has been acting strangely. The key is to be observant and willing to experiment a bit to find the magic combination.

When Lynne had trouble getting to and staying asleep, before I discovered what white noise could do and after I had played all the music she enjoyed, I used an antique metronome that belonged to Lynne's mother. The ticking of the metronome helped Lynne to relax and sleep better once I got her to start focusing on the ticking noise and think of nothing else. It was noisy! It could be heard several rooms away. I put it in our walk-in closet to keep the noise from being disturbing.

If you are not familiar with the concept of white noise, in a nutshell, it is a sound that makes other sounds seem to disappear. Quite often, parents will use white noise to mask unwanted noises and help newborns sleep better. At one point, I used a white noise machine that I found in an online baby catalog. The upside was that it helped mask the outside noises, which would help Lynne relax and sleep better. The downside is that I am now on every baby or child catalog and magazine mailing list in the country. An additional downside was, after about six months, the noise started to bother Lynne when she could no longer figure out what the various noises were or where the sounds were coming from. So now it lives in our closet in case I may want to use it again in the future.

For many years, Lynne would say she was solar-powered. As I look back, I can see how the various office environments she worked in, and their exposure to sunlight did make a difference in her overall attitude. When she worked in a basement, she tended to be less like herself than when she worked in the sunny upstairs office.

Lynne has developed what I call "cloudy day syndrome." This is a term I made up to describe how withdrawn Lynne becomes on cloudy days. The answer to the cloudy day syndrome and her solar power needs was to buy artificial daylight lights and have them on during cloudy days to give her the impression that it is sunny. I cannot tell you what light wavelengths do, but when we have a cloudy day, I try to mimic the sun by turning these daylights on and off as the day progresses. I am likely just fooling myself, but it does seem to help Lynne with her cloudy day syndrome to some degree.

But this is Alzheimer's disease, and I have found that there are certain times of the year, when the sun is at its lowest point in the sky; Lynne receives too much exposure to the sun. For these few weeks, I bring out the blackout curtains to control the amount of sunlight she gets.

Something I discovered in year ten was the impact of the television on Lynne. While she is usually not able to focus on the screen, she is still able to hear and understand what is being said. She will occasionally laugh at something said; when the actors are arguing or making too much noise, she might cover her ears or say *"Shh,"* thinking the actors are in the room with her.

One day, Lynne was listening to a show, and something said on the show upset her. I assumed she again thought the people on the TV show were in the room with her. She was very withdrawn and quiet. (I know she is aphasic, but you get the idea.) This lasted for most of three days, and of course, I could not find the right questions to get the answers. But after quizzing her and eliminating various possibilities, I was able to put her mind at ease once I determined the television was the likely culprit and not something I said or did. So now I am very selective about the shows she is exposed to. This is just another example of how this caregiving business is an ever-changing learning experience and demonstrates the need for environmental controls.

While we are on the subject of television and comforting the sick, I ran across something strictly by accident. (Remember, we learn as we go in this caregiving job.) In the good old days, Lynne and I vacationed in Vermont two or three times a year for over ten years. The only television available was through an air antenna, so our choices were limited. And after having missed out on a few major events while vacationing in the past, we would watch the news and then Regis and Kathie Lee. We didn't want to be surprised or shocked because we were once again off the grid, so this became our standard bill of fare while on vacation.

I felt that going back to something familiar might remind Lynne of the good old days, so one day; I parked her in front of Regis and Kelly. It took her a few days, but she eventually remembered watching Regis and Kathie Lee when we were in Vermont. But something else happened. This station started broadcasting Rachael Ray's show after Regis and Kelly. Lynne's reaction to Rachael Ray was instantaneous and so positive that she rarely misses an episode. I even had to DVR some for the weekends so Lynne would have her Rachael. I have not been able to determine what made this instant connection. I assume it's the voice, since Lynne usually remembered people by their accents, speech patterns, word choice, and the like. I do know it is not visual, since Lynne rarely looks at the television screen. But whatever it is, we have at least one Rachael Ray viewing most every day.

Delusions and Hallucinations

Irst, there can be a fine line between delusions and hallucinations. Delusions are false or mistaken beliefs or ideas about something tangible. Hallucinations are things that somebody imagines sensing that are not present or actually occurring at the time.

Most all caregivers agree that when dealing with a dementia patient's delusions and hallucinations, you should just go with it, and hopefully it will pass. If you make a big deal out of them, all you will accomplish is creating another problem that has no upside for either of you, and most likely, both parties will lose out.

Before my mother relocated to Happy Valley, the only event I would consider a hallucination would be the numerous telephone calls she received from my grandmother. She was so convincing when talking about these calls that if I didn't know better, I would swear she was actually receiving these calls. I would tell her that her mother had passed away many years ago, so she could not have made these calls. At times, I would challenge these calls by showing her a copy of my grandmother's obituary. Undaunted, my mother would continue to insist that she received these calls.

While my mother was at Happy Valley, she was always in the wrong place, having been kidnapped by a list of bad guys. Every day—sometimes multiple times a day—she was planning to escape when the guards weren't watching. She would quite often vocally and aggressively demand her freedom, which was often accompanied by threats of violence against the staff.

After convincing her that she had not been kidnapped but instead was there for her health, I would tell her we had to talk to the front desk about the checkout procedures, so no escape was necessary. Another way of handling it was to tell her that she needed to stay until the doctor could check her out. Telling her that the doctor visit was free usually won the day because it never hurts to get something for free, especially from a doctor.

The bottom line is that you must work with the situation without irritating anybody. And take heart; the probability of the situation and your response being remembered tomorrow is slim at best. Unfortunately, most delusions and hallucinations are recurring, so be prepared. The test of a true caregiver is keeping a straight face when the victim's delusions and hallucinations become outrageous in your mind.

When dealing with my mother's delusions, before she went to Happy Valley, it was important for me (and maybe it was just me) to understand the basis for her delusions. Early on, her delusions quite frankly surprised or confused me. Understanding the source of some of her delusions assisted me in defusing or deflecting them.

In order to be prepared for an AD victim's delusions and hallucinations, you need to do a bit of research to be better prepared to help your loved one. Try to get your demented loved one to talk to you calmly. You in turn should respond as patiently as possible without challenging, correcting, interjecting, or ridiculing about what they are experiencing. Your job is to determine how you can help in the situation, not to convince your AD victim that they are mistaken in their understanding of the situation or are seeing or hearing things that are not there.

When your AD victim is as calm and rational as possible, try to talk about the general subject of their delusions and hallucinations. Just do not make the mistake of searching for details too quickly. You need to skirt around the edges at first until you can gather enough bits and pieces of information to talk about it when your loved one is "normal." The key is to sniff around until you feel that they would not mind talking about whatever is bothering them. You may want to enlist other family members or friends to retrieve the information if your loved one is not comfortable talking with you about it. Your mission is to determine what the problem is, determine the possible answer, and not dwell on it. But take care not to push too hard or too fast for the answers. It may take months to find your way through this minefield.

I had success in dealing with my mother when I let her do the talking or ranting, no matter how strange or aggressive it became. It made me better able to figure out how to calm her down and let her know that I was there to help her. Remember, too much talking on your part could be perceived as a challenge, and the groundwork that you are trying to lay or maintain could all be destroyed by over-talking the situation.

I have often used the line that AD victims are sick, not stupid. Yes, they have issues with memory and decision-making skills. But you still need to take your delusion- and hallucination-busting stories for a test drive because the chances of their recurring are very likely, and you may find the right combination of words or techniques to diffuse the situation before it truly gets out of hand.

I think my grandparents had my mother's piano from her childhood piano lessons until they moved into their single-wide trailer in 1965, where there was certainly not enough room for a piano. What actually happened to the piano remains a mystery to this day. This mystery kept my mother on edge for a few years, especially during her sundowning. But she was determined to discover what happened to the piano and retrieve it so she could continue taking lessons and start playing again. While I vaguely remember a piano in the front room of one of my grandparents' homes, I never saw my mother play a musical instrument of any description.

My story of what happened to this mysterious, vanishing piano developed over several months. When she started asking and then demanding to know what happened to her piano, my responses began with, "I don't remember a piano." Then I said, "I think they gave the piano to Cousin Clara because her daughter was taking piano lessons, and they couldn't afford to buy a piano." This evolved into, "I think they donated it to a church." None of these responses were acceptable to my mother because Cousin Clara had her own piano or why would they give her piano to a church, and which church was it?

Undaunted, I continued to develop a palatable story that could not be challenged but at the same time sounded believable. Eventually, I came up with, "When they decided to move from the house across from the high school, they donated your piano to the music department of the high school so that the piano would get used. Since they did not have enough space in the smaller house and you did not want to bear the expense of having it moved from North Carolina to Virginia, the piano went to the high school." This falls in the category of not letting the facts get in the way of a good lie in order to quash a delusion. Also make sure your story has enough details to make it sound like the truth. In this case, there was some truth to my story. My grandparents had lived across from the high school and did, in fact, move to a smaller house at some point in time.

When my mother wished to contact the school to check on the status of her piano, I informed her that the principal of the school and the director of the music program so many years ago had long since retired and most likely had expired. I did not tell her that the high school was gutted by fire, which would have naturally destroyed her mysterious piano.

Sundowning

In the early stages of my mother's Alzheimer's, in addition to the short-term memory loss and the loss of some executive functions, she started sundowning. If you are not familiar with the term, it is a temporary cognitive downturn that typically occurs in the late afternoon or early evening.

My mother's sundowning episodes happened every day and would last for about two hours. As quick as these episodes came on, they would be gone, and she would be back to her version of normal. When my mother started sundowning, it was a little upsetting, especially since I did not really understand what was happening until I spoke with others who had witnessed sundowning in other dementia patients. I certainly could not call my mother's doctor, the one who could or would not say Alzheimer's or dementia. So once I had the term sundowning and a general idea of what was I dealing with, I went to the Internet again to do research so I would be better prepared for this scheduled silliness.

My mother was generally passive when she reached her golden years until the sundowning took over. Every afternoon she was sundowning. It was full throttle, and often nothing would stop her, calm her, or defuse her until it ran its course. It was so consistent that you could nearly set your watch by her. While in general, she was never physically aggressive, she became much more verbally demanding, more confused about time and location, and agitated by the least little thing—and then would come the telephone calls from my dead grandmother.

After Mom moved to Happy Valley, I timed my visits for the sundowning hours so she would be less of a disruption to the staff and residents. Even though she seldom knew me, my presence tended to redirect her, calm her, and keep her entertained. For the most part, it did help, but it sometimes put me in awkward situations, especially the day she thought I was her husband. Had the nurse not come by to ask a question, I know nothing would have happened except some very hurt feelings and more confusion.

Lynne's sundowning, as you might expect, is different. She is nearly as consistent as my mother was in time and duration but with two obvious differences. During the middle stages of the disease, she stopped sundowning during the winter months. Lynne's sundowning starts about 3:30 p.m. and goes until about 6:00 p.m., plus or minus thirty minutes on either end. And unlike my mother's agitation, Lynne is just plain restless. During the middle stages of the disease, if she were lying down, she would get up every ten to fifteen minutes. Often, even if she was lying in bed, she would get up, come to me, and tell me she wanted to go to bed. And there were also requests on occasion to go home. I would tell her, as calmly as possible and as many times as necessary, that she was in bed or at home. After several times of asking to go to bed, go home, or both, she would give up and just go back to her bed in her home and take a nap.

When Lynne entered the later stages of AD, her sundowning became more of a wandering, standing, and staring sort of thing that was punctuated with the very occasional request for home or bed. The upside is that she's getting a little exercise, but of course, there is the downside. (Remember, this is Alzheimer's, so there's almost always a downside for every upside.) Her already limited vision becomes more limited while she is sundowning, so tripping over furniture or the occasional pet or bumping into closed doors is a real possibility. The pets that sleep pretty much anywhere they want usually find themselves in the walkway. So in order to keep Lynne from tripping over a sleeping dog or cat, I make a general announcement, "Mom is on the move." This usually gives them enough warning to move out of the way or move to higher ground.

Activities of Daily Living

As time goes on, just like the victim and the disease itself, we caregivers go through stages. We increase our involvement in the daily activities of our loved one, get less sleep, and worry more about whether we are doing everything we can, and try desperately to find more quality time in the time we have left together.

This, of course, brings us to the dreaded ADLs—Activities of Daily Living. For new caregivers, ADLs are simply what they sound like—dressing, hygiene, bowel and bladder elimination, medication management, transportation, and anything else a typical adult does on a daily basis to satisfy the basics of living an ordinary life. To get a small idea of what is in store for you as the disease takes over more and more, keep a detailed notebook for a normal day of your regular activities. It is amazing just how many things we do every day without thinking about the mechanics of something as simple as eating a meal, getting dressed, or using the bathroom.

When I signed on for the care of my wife, I assumed there would come a time that I would be responsible for her feeding, dressing, and hygiene. I was confident that I could meet the challenge and felt comfortable with doing Lynne's ADLs. I was also confident that I could possibly meet some resistance when the time came for me to step in. Of course, the question is always—when and how do you start taking over the ADLs? In my case, I didn't ask permission to help; I just helped. I'm just that kind of guy!

When did I start feeding? It was simple. When the dog started gaining weight and Lynne's shirt and pants started looking like she had been in a food fight, I knew it was time.

The first assistance I gave was cutting her food into manageable sizes. As time went on, I would help her chase down the last few veggies on her plate to help her finish eating her meal. Eventually that gave way to feeding her everything that required a utensil. For quite a while, she was still able handle finger foods with some occasional assistance, but eventually, all of her feeding was up to me. The upsides were—the dog lost weight, and I had less laundry to do.

It is tempting to cut corners with food selection for your AD victim and opt for soup, sandwiches, and frozen dinners. But be mindful of the nutrition that you are providing. High levels of fat, sodium, and carbohydrates are not good for anybody, least of all the sick. Also be observant of your victim's post-meal actions. I found that with Lynne, too many carbohydrates caused her to become more sullen. Since I am diabetic, I was able to cook for both of us using diabetes-oriented menus. That's not to say that we don't occasionally have pizza, French fries, and the like, but as they taught us at the Diabetes Education Center—everything in moderation.

Some caregivers prepare the AD victim's meals separate from their own meals, choosing to play short-order cook and to avoid exposing other family members to the sometimes challenging eating process if they have to feed the victim and the victim doesn't want to cooperate.

While on the subject of food and nutrition, here are few words on the meal replacement shakes. They are tasty and convenient, to be sure, but for some folks, they can be tough on the budget. Also the AD victim may not like the taste or might object to being fed "old people" food. Take the meal replacement shake nutrition information to your local vitamin store or the vitamin counter at the drug store, and do a little nutrition comparison shopping for a product called whey protein. (There are other varieties, but whey is my preference.) Then swing into the grocery store, and locate the breakfast powders that you mix with milk. There are many upsides to this dietary chemistry experiment. You can control the amounts, usually lower the costs, vary the flavor, and use something other than cow's milk if that's a concern. And if your AD victim is having bowel problems, you can add some of the unflavored fiber.

Hydration is very important. Whenever my cognitively challenged loved ones did not get enough water, I could see it in their functionality. No matter how many times I asked or told the Happy Valley staff to make sure my mother stayed hydrated, they rarely took a moment to offer her any water from the stash of the bottled water in her room that I knew she would drink. Lynne gets a cup of water first thing in the morning with her meds. At least twice during the day and at night with her pills, she drinks more water. Water is good for what ails you—inside and out.

While we are in the water department, there may come a time where your AD victim may exhibit a problem with dysphagia (difficulties with swallowing). Normally, the first time you see this problem with swallowing will be with thinner liquids, like water. Drop by the drug store, and look or ask for a product called Thick-It. Just add a bit to whatever he or she is eating or drinking, and it should resolve the problem—at least for a while.

Helping Lynne dress was also based on her declining abilities. (Duh!) Granted, we had a lot of experience over the years undressing each other, but seldom did we reverse the process. As Lynne started to fumble with buttons, zippers, and shoelaces, I would step in and help. Buttons, zippers, and shoelaces of course gave way to helping her put on her pants the right way because it would take her a full ten minutes to do it wrong, or she would just give up in frustration. Putting on a shirt was pretty much the same—backward, inside out, and, my personal favorite, trying to put her head through the armhole of a T-shirt. Shoes and socks were the last obstacle. There were not as many options, so there was a much lower failure rate. But eventually, just like with eating, I became her personal valet.

We did have a little trouble with toileting, since Lynne, like most everybody, did not want an audience while sitting on the toilet. So I would escort her to the bathroom, get her situated, and excuse myself with an "I'll be back in a minute or two" and then quietly stand out of sight in the hallway, waiting for the customary noises. Then I would "return" after announcing myself, using a soft voice so she would feel I was coming back from somewhere away from the bathroom.

Eventually, I did have to remain in the bathroom when Lynne's balance and her myoclonus became an issue. I explained to her several times that I was afraid she might fall, so I had to stay. I would just stand with my back to her so I would not make her uncomfortable because I was watching her. In reality, I was watching her in the mirror. But what she didn't know would not disrupt the call of nature.

Showering eventually became an issue. In the early days, we would just shower together like we had so many times before the Alzheimer's—just without the sexual component, usually. After a while, I introduced the shower stool, which for the most part, worked well once I got Lynne into the tub.

The stool was replaced by a sliding/swiveling shower bench when Lynne's balance became an issue, even though she would still be okay standing in the tub. Standing on one foot while stepping over the side of the tub became a danger. The bench works well, although she does not like the plastic seat or the loss of control when the seat is moving. I like it, as it makes the showering easier because you can position your victim in the right place to do the job without a lot of lifting, stretching, or body contortions.

We had fairly smooth transitions on nearly everything related to hygiene when it came to my taking over Lynne's ADLs. But one thing that escaped me for quite a while. No matter how hard I tried, I just could not seem to find the magic combination for brushing Lynne's teeth. Second-party oral hygiene for an Alzheimer's victim is difficult at best unless you are a dentist or hygienist with the experience, tools, and chair to do the job.

We had multiple issues in simply trying to brush Lynne's teeth. First, there is the sixteen-inch difference in our heights, so the angle of attack was the first thing we had to overcome. After getting the height difference ironed out, there was the problem of Lynne keeping her mouth open enough but not too much. She also always wants to bite the toothbrush. We started with the electric toothbrush that we had been using for years, then a regular adult toothbrush, a kid's toothbrush, and finally, a little fingertip brush. All would work to a certain degree, for a while, but eventually, all would fail. I asked for advice from my hygienist, which yielded no better ideas.

Then I discovered little sponges on a stick. They look a bit like a sponge lollipop. This certainly is not the greatest in tooth brushing technology, but it is better than nothing. I found small ones online that were adequate—but barely. When I mentioned them to the hospice nurse, she supplied me with another brand of these little sponge lollipops. The sponge was a bit larger and the stick a bit longer and stronger than the ones I had used previously.

Once we got the angle of attack figured out, implements to do the job effectively, and had developed a routine that was yielding fairly consistent positive results, Lynne changed the field of play. She started standing or sitting with her head tilted so far forward that I had to practically stand on my head to see what I was doing. So that's when I developed the hair-pull technique.

Lynne began letting her hair grow long about fifteen years ago, and I frankly do not have the heart to cut it to make her hair care easier on both of us. But the long hair comes in handy when brushing her teeth. In order to keep her stable and keep her head from dropping down, making it more difficult to find her mouth and brush her teeth, I simply wrap her ponytail around my hand and keep enough tension on her hair while holding on to her neck or shoulder. This is not a perfect way to approach oral hygiene, but I don't have the luxury of a dentist chair and saliva ejector in my bathroom.

Alzheimer's Assisted Living Facilities

I know this book is all about caregiving at home. So why am I writing about checking out assisted living facilities? In case you have not determined the obvious, stuff can happen that is beyond your control that can get in the way of the lofty goal of taking care of your loved one at home until the end. Since you are a human being, you can get sick, injured, or dead; the home you are using can become uninhabitable by fire, acts of nature, or foreclosure; you may have to, like me, choose between two people; or you may just be too burned out and unable to face another day of caring for your loved one. There is no shame in the latter. Caregiving is a long, arduous process, and there should no embarrassment on your part in admitting defeat by a disease that has claimed millions of victims and caregivers.

So here are a few personal observations about assisted living facilities and what to watch out for. First, not all assisted living facilities are able to care for Alzheimer's patients. Before you start the process of determining which facilities you wish to visit, make sure they accept AD patients.

Before I get into the nuts and bolts of putting your loved one into "The Home", I must clear up one of the common mistakes that many caregivers and family members make—the possibility that your demented loved one will want to move into any care facility. It occasionally does happen, but don't hold your breath unless blue is your best color.

Just like making funeral arrangements, you need to go to these facilities with your eyes wide open. Don't have preconceived ideas, and be willing to ask a ton of questions while keeping your hand firmly planted on your wallet. It is no secret that the price of getting old or ill and needing a place to live is quite expensive. It is not only expensive in the wallet, but also very expensive to the physical and mental well-being of a dementia patient and his or her family members.

So, let's tackle the costs up front. The national average is roughly $3,000 per month. That is just a rough estimate, not considering the room type, ups and extras, locality, or anything else. The price of my mother's stay at Happy Valley was nearly three times the national average, which did not include medications, diapers, special event fees, furniture I purchased for the room, and all the lost odds and ends (usually clothing) I had to replace. Unless your AD victim has insurance that covers long-term care that monthly fee is coming from you. Medicare, Medicaid, and customary health insurance do not cover assisted living or Alzheimer's assisted living. Believe me, *"Ouch"* does not even begin to describe years of costs for living in these types of facilities.

When we determined my mother would have to enter assisted living, Lynne and I visited four different facilities based on a list I received from an elder housing placement agency at no charge. (*www.aplaceformom.com*) This extremely long list included large facilities and group homes. As a starting point, based on the geographic locations and a rating system, we chose two of each and went for an interview and a tour.

Group homes, while good for some, certainly would not have worked in my mother's case. These facilities are for the patient who tends to be easier to manage, is not prone to outbursts, and is not liable to wander. The two group homes we visited were homes within the community. The first was a 1970s three-bedroom house stuck in the middle of a large subdivision. The second place was a mini-mansion built in a very expensive part of the county. To say the two houses were drastically different is an understatement.

A friend of ours, whose father lived in an Alzheimer's group home for a number of years, was quite satisfied with the services provided and the environment that he lived in until his death. While we appreciated her input, I was a bit skeptical before going in. But whether the ideal place was a group home or a full-size regular facility, the important thing was to do what was best for my mother, whether it was going to be for the long run or for a few months while we made the modifications required to my house so she could move in with us.

The two group homes we chose to visit were chosen very much at random from approximately fifteen that met our location and rating requirements. We were concerned with the distance, as Lynne and I would be visiting every day. We wanted to avoid driving long distances in the often congested Washington, DC-area traffic.

Upon meeting with the management and staff of the two group homes, Lynne and I made a list of the more obvious defects, which included:

- Very small staff—usually only one person on duty (but to be fair, the homes were only set up for two or three residents). As we all find out, one dementia patient can be a handful for one caregiver. One of the homes was managed and staffed solely by a seventy-year-old woman. She was a nice lady, but I just could not image her handling multiple AD victims.

- A lack of security—one home didn't even have a deadbolt on any door or any alarm or security system. This not only made it easier for wanderers to get out, but also helped any bad guys have an easier way in.

- One home had a fence that was strictly for decoration, not detention. This particular house was very close to two major highways. The other facility had a rusty, three-foot-high chain link fence—certainly not decorative and just slightly functional.

- Numerous slip and fall hazards—both places used a lot of tile or laminate flooring, making it easier for the staff to keep the floors clean. But these floor coverings are definitely a slip or fall hazard.

- One home used a detached two-car garage for its activity room, and there was no fencing between the house and the garage to keep a potential wanderer from disappearing.
- The fees were comparable to the full-size, regular facilities, even though the group homes apparently fell far short with what they had to offer.

Don't get me wrong; group homes can be great alternatives to the large, sometimes impersonal facilities. We chose these two group homes strictly at random off the list the agency provided and determined they were less than ideal for my mother's situation.

In looking at the full-size, regular facilities, keep in mind that your loved one will be part of the crowd. While the facility will have your person's best interests in mind, they sometimes have to temper one person's wants or needs against those of the larger group—and of course, the corporate image and the bottom line.

In our comparison of the big name regular facilities, we chose one large and one small facility. The large facility had multiple floors and a population of approximately 150 assisted living and dementia residents. The second facility was one level and had a total population of approximately sixty residents with fifteen to eighteen being Alzheimer's or dementia patients. Both facilities were part of the same corporation. One was owned by the corporation; the other facility was owned by the local hospital and was managed by this organization.

The larger of the two facilities was quite plush. It looked and felt like a high-end hotel, not an old folks home—and certainly not a dementia facility. Even the dementia floor was well decorated and quite comfortable, with a variety of room layouts and sizes. I would have been quite comfortable living in either part of this facility. The place was clean, well staffed, and quite inviting. It was certainly not as low-key as the group homes. It was truly a place I felt my mother would be comfortable, safe, and well cared for.

The last facility we reviewed, the one we ultimately chose, offered much the same as the larger facility. But what tipped the scales was that it seemed more like a family. It was not as big and certainly not as decorated, but it looked like my mother's home and lifestyle. It was clean and well-staffed; it certainly had a smaller resident population, and the rooms were all fairly standard, but the whole package just screamed, "Hazel lives here"—which she did for about two and a half years.

When making the big decision, no matter the type and size of the facility, don't make the mistakes that many families have made in selecting a new home for your AD loved one by making assumptions. Proceed with caution.

- Above all else, ask a lot of questions of the facility manager—and, if possible, staff members—and take detailed notes. This is a huge decision that will affect you and your family, and most importantly, your cognitively challenged loved one.

- Do not make the decision on your first visit unless you absolutely have to based on events at home. If you need to move quickly, remember that the number of people moving into and out of these facilities affects the availability of rooms.

- Take time to do your homework on the facilities that you feel will be a good fit for your loved one. In making this decision, understand that the more questions you ask, the more likely you will be happy with your decision—at least from the business standpoint.

- Talk to the facility coordinators about specific concerns. Even ask for another walk-through if you need to clarify anything. The facility coordinators know this is a big financial decision for you as well as an emotional one. This is the stage where there are no stupid questions. But listen closely to the answers because they can be vague generalities that may make you think you are getting what you are paying for and that your loved one will be truly content.

There are many factors to consider when determining your loved one's future home. Get the details on any concerns you have about the facility and how your loved one will fit in, be cared for, and be kept safe. For us, with my mother's history of wandering, we were interested in an explanation of the equipment the facilities used to discourage and prevent wandering. If a resident escaped, we wanted to know what procedures were in place to retrieve the wanderer. I was also interested to discover what emergency evacuation procedures were in place in case of fire or natural disaster. Since we were so close to Washington, DC, we wanted to know how the facilities were prepared should another terrorist attack occur. You may or may not have these same concerns, but the key is to get the answers to any questions or concerns before signing the bottom line.

As I was leaving Happy Valley one evening, a couple about my age was sitting on the front porch. I assumed they were visiting one of the residents. They started asking questions about the facility, the staff, and how well I felt my mother was being cared for. I was quick to give them the answers they were seeking after I determined who they were and why they were asking all the questions. While I did have a few small complaints and concerns, I was generally satisfied with the staff and the care they were providing.

The couple was visiting some of the facilities around the area for the man's wife, who was Early Onset. The woman with him was his sister, who was helping in the wife's care. We spoke for about twenty minutes about my experience with the facility and the staff, the strong suits, the shortfalls, and the things I felt could have been done better. A few days later, their very special person moved into the facility. She was a joy, and nearly every day when I visited my mother, this very special person greeted me with a big smile. I could not help but wonder who she was before the Alzheimer's took her away from her loving family. When I returned to the facility to clean out my mother's room, I found out that this very special person had passed away. Even though I did not know her before the AD took her away, I was saddened by her passing.

Somebody will be writing a very large check every month. Make sure you know what you are paying for, and make sure you get absolutely everything in writing. "All inclusive" usually is not, and "à la carte" means you will get a bill for every little thing. I spoke with a family member of a resident at Happy Valley about the facility his loved one was in previously. He told me that the à la carte monthly bill was many pages long, as the facility listed every single item individually.

This is not an indictment of all facilities, but there have been instances of abuse involving dementia patients because of their inability to defend themselves or identify who victimized them, whether the wrongdoer was a staff member, another patient, or a visitor. Once you have gone to the facilities to interview the staff and check them out with a physical walk-through, contact the state or local agencies responsible for nursing homes and assisted living facilities to determine if they have a rap sheet. Keep in mind that some states have a different set of regulatory guidelines or oversight offices for assisted living facilities, as they are different from nursing homes, rehabilitation centers, and hospitals. But do the homework so you are not surprised.

Yes, your loved one is moving into a new home, and you want them to feel like they are still in their own home. When moving them into their new home, you (or your AD loved one) will likely want to have personal items that will help make the new surroundings more familiar to increase their level of comfort and calm. Some families treat the room like a total move-in, while others go with just the basics.

- Leave the irreplaceable and breakable items at home. Things have a way of getting lost or being mishandled in this environment.

- Mark everything with your loved one's name, but be assured that all the marks in the world will not insure that any items will be safely returned.
- The staff may not take the best care of clothing and furnishings. Consider the possibility of damage from cleaning and disinfectant products. I have no idea what they spray on everything during a scabies outbreak, but it's sticky and can stain.
- Be prepared for glasses, hearing aids, dentures, and the like to disappear. When my mother moved into Happy Valley, her glasses disappeared on the third day.

Many times, I told the facility managers, the dementia coordinators, and the staff members at Happy Valley that in order for us to all be on the same page in caring for my mother, they needed to maintain a line of communication, and I would reciprocate. Their idea of communication was quick chats in the hallway. To them, the better care plan was to keep my mother medicated enough so she would not be a bother, but still be functional enough to take care of herself to a certain degree.

After seeing the drug cabinet for the fifteen to eighteen dementia residents, I am quite sure my mother was not the only one being quieted. But in the entire time my mother was a resident at this facility, the lines of communication were quite often disrupted, and the staff members still relied on ambush communications. With the large turnover in front office staff, no sooner would I find a staff member that would work with me than he or she would be shuffled out only to be replaced by someone with a closed-door and closed-mouth policy.

"Sarah," an Alzheimer's patient, was a resident in an AD facility that had very little security and no wandering prevention devices more than door locks and staff watching. It seemed that Sarah did not care much for the accommodations, so several times a week, she would leave the facility. She usually got no more than a few blocks away, so her recovery was usually quick and uneventful. The family tired of the facility constantly misplacing their loved one, so they decided to move Sarah to another AD facility with better security.

Two of Sarah's children, "Debbie" and "Bob," were going to the facility to give the required thirty-day notice of Sarah's move and to start planning the move. As they sat at a traffic light, Debbie and Bob were discussing the logistics of the move and Mom's possible reaction. As they sat talking, Bob spotted Sarah walking down the sidewalk alongside the very busy highway nearly a mile from the facility. Debbie made a U-turn, and as they pulled up by Sarah, Bob asked her if she wanted a ride home. Sarah thanked him and got in the car for her ride home. The facility decided that it would waive the thirty-day notice, as the family retrieved Sarah and the staff had no idea that she was out of the building again.

Adult diapers supplied by the facility are the ultimate profit center. When my mother was at Happy Valley, the daily fee for the diaper service was the same as a single package of thirty diapers bought on sale at a local department store. For my mother, who usually used one diaper per day, the math was simple—about $9 for a thirty-count package of brand X adult diapers versus the facility-supplied brand X variety at $9 per day. The difference was over $250 per month. The fee that was charged by the facility also supposedly included gloves, cleaning supplies, lotions, and the like. In my desire to not go broke on diapers and other essentials, I procured the cleaning supplies and lotions from the same store as the diapers. Then went to the warehouse store and found a better quality glove and enough cleaning supplies to more than fulfill Happy Valley's cleanliness needs.

If you take nothing away from this little primer on senior housing, take this. If you plan to visit anyone at an AD facility, do not take your germs into a closed community, such as a nursing home or assisted living facility. If you are sick, no matter how badly you want to visit, you have to stay away. All it takes is one sick outsider, and the residents start dropping like flies. So just keep your germs at home where they belong. Bottom line—don't be a problem.

But also know about scabies. If you have had scabies, you know it. If you have not had it or are unfamiliar with it, jump on the Internet to get to know the warning signs. It's the itch that just keeps on giving, and the treatment is no walk in the park either.

A scabies outbreak in a closed community will often cause the community to be closed to the public until it is cleared by the Health Department or similar authority. Try explaining to your loved one why he or she is itching and that you haven't been there for several days because of the itch that just keeps on giving.

The situation of putting your loved one into a facility is never easy, and it never gets easier. In my travels in reviewing the four different facilities as well as times I have visited other facilities, I have noticed not one of them has the words "Fun House" on the front door. When making the decision involving placing your loved one in a facility, remember that this is not going to be easy, fun, inexpensive, or forgettable. And that is just your side of the story. Just imagine the panic or hatred that is going through your loved one's mind when you drive out of sight.

Hospice Care

No matter how well you care for your loved one, eventually the end will be in sight, and that's where hospice comes in. Hospice has a bit of a bad reputation; to many, it is usually known as the Grim Reaper. Understand that the first qualifier for hospice is that the doctor feels that death is imminent—within six months. That does not mean that six months after entering hospice care your loved one's story will be over. I know this, since Lynne has been in hospice for over two years at the time of this writing. There was a 101-year-old dementia resident at Happy Valley, who had been under hospice care for approximately nine months and lived to tell about it three years later. So hospice does not necessarily mean the end.

Placing your loved one into hospice does not mean that anybody is giving up on your loved one. Hospice is not in a position of controlling you or your loved one. The service hospice provides is an extension of the caregiving effort. Many people are under the impression that hospice comes in, hooks up the morphine, and puts people to sleep. This is a very common misconception. In fact, patients in hospice care can still have treatments available to them for managing the symptoms associated with their disease.

Hospice is a team-oriented approach that addresses the medical, physical, emotional, and spiritual needs of the patient as well as providing support to the family. The care hospice provides is palliative, which means that hospice workers are more concerned with pain and other symptoms than seeking to cure.

Studies have shown that palliative care is good medicine, since it can enhance the quality of life, which can help patients live longer.

Studies have shown that people in hospice care can actually live months longer, suffer less from depression, and have a better quality of life.

Our hospice team is comprised of a physician, a nurse practitioner, a registered nurse, a licensed practical nurse, a social worker, a nondenominational chaplain, and various staff nurses and volunteers who call to inquire about patient and caregiver condition as well as medication or equipment needs. Any medication or equipment used in connection with the hospice effort comes at no charge to you (after any deductibles and co-payments), as does any face time with the medical staff, social worker, and chaplain. Medicare, Medicaid, or your insurance covers the costs. If you have no insurance, then your bank account will require hospice care.

Since hospice is part of the care plan, your doctors are still involved in your loved one's care. The patient remains at home, and you will still remain the primary caregiver, so you will still have input on everything. And unlike most doctors, hospice is available twenty-four hours a day. There is always somebody available to discuss or resolve emergent problems, including riding to the rescue at four o'clock in the morning. It is like the good old days when the family doctor was always available with a telephone call.

Lynne is currently under hospice care, which is paid for by Medicare. It looks to be of limited value in the grand scheme of things. But it is reassuring for me to know that a qualified, experienced medical professional is coming to our house every week to check Lynne's vitals, her overall health, and how the disease is progressing. Then there is the safety net of having around-the-clock emergency response just a telephone call away if the wheels fall off the wagon.

Late in year eleven, Lynne's hospice nurse and I noticed a change in Lynne's facial features and her body language. Instead of her usual vacant stare, Lynne looked like she was mad about something. And while she normally sat slightly bent forward at the waist, she was leaning so far forward she looked as if she was folded in half.

Although Lynne had never shown signs of depression, the hospice team, Lynne's neurologist's staff, and I discussed the possibility of depression. Since Lynne's Alzheimer's symptoms were unusual, I felt her symptoms of depression might also be different. So, after talking and thinking about these changes, we all agreed to start Lynne on an antidepressant early in year twelve.

After a week on medication, Lynne's sour look eased, her posture improved, and she started sleeping better. So hospice is not the end of possibilities; it can be an opportunity for improvement.

Even though Lynne's hospice nurse visits us once a week, I receive a call from a staff nurse every evening. Any information I give to the evening nurse is entered into Lynne's file so the regular visiting nurse is kept apprised of any changes. Each evening nurse is not only knowledgeable but wonderful to talk with, and I look forward to their daily calls.

Could I check Lynne's vital signs and contact the neurologist's office directly with any changes or trot her out to primary care for checkups and emergent changes? Of course I could. I did it before hospice came along, and if hospice goes away because of Lynne's inability to be recertified, I can do it again. But I also know that as Lynne starts to fade away, the level of hospice involvement will increase until, if necessary, they have to hook up the morphine and let her slip away.

Clinical Trials

When we received Lynne's diagnosis from the doctor who finally ran the right test, I asked him, while Lynne sat sobbing at finally receiving the diagnosis so long in coming, "What do we do now, since we finally know what we are facing?" His response was, "You should look into clinical trials. If you find anything that looks promising; send me the information, and I will decide whether you should proceed." There certainly were a lot of "you's" in that guidance. I had no formal medical training except searching the Internet and a high school first aid class. I was supposed to interpret the clinical trial code and decide what trials Lynne and I should look into?

A few days after receiving the diagnosis, Lynne and I discussed participating in clinical trials. We discussed the upsides and downsides and everything that needed to be considered before entering into the unknown of the clinical trial business from the patient's point of view. We also had to determine how we would cover my mother while we were away from the house.

I located a website (*www.clinicaltrials.gov*) that listed every clinical trial and searched it for any AD trial that Lynne could qualify for immediately so we would not lose any more time than necessary. One of the qualifiers is usually the trial candidate's MMSE score. We did not want to run the risk of Lynne's score going down too much before finding a trial. One of the factors that often eliminated Lynne was that since she had just been diagnosed and just started taking her AD medication, she would not qualify, since many of the trials wanted the patient on medication for several months at a minimum or not on medication for a period of time.

My first attempt to get Lynne into a trial was not successful. I contacted a university medical center in New York that was recruiting for a trial. Lynne was qualified, and we only needed to be at the test site once a week. Since neither of us was working, and I felt confident we could get coverage for my mother and the pets while we made the weekly trip, I contacted the trial coordinator. While they were interested because of Lynne's unique symptoms, their main concern was the possibility of us not being able to make the trip during the winter months. I am sure the possibility of side effects, especially en route, was also a concern with us so living far from the test site.

After locating another trial that looked promising and discussing it with Lynne's neurologist, I contacted Georgetown University Medical Center Memory Disorders Program via e-mail and received a telephone call back less than an hour later. The woman at Georgetown asked some basic questions about Lynne's Alzheimer's and her overall health. That call generated a call from a nurse practitioner—the trial coordinator—who asked more direct questions. The most important question focused on Lynne's ability to understand what the trials involved, if she understood the possibly of side effects, and if she was prepared for any type of side effect.

Since I had been doing all of the talking, I put Lynne on the telephone, and the coordinator asked her straight out if she understood the possibility of side effects and if she was sure that she wanted to participate in a clinical trial. Lynne answered her directly with, "What good is a fatal disease if you can't make use of it?" We started in a Phase II clinical trial a few months later after Lynne had been on her AD medications for the prescribed time stated in the trial protocol. This turned out to be a different trial than the one I had initially contacted them about.

Clinical trials include testing of new and existing drugs, therapies, diagnostic procedures, and medical equipment. Needless to say, clinical trials are an important part of conquering any disease—especially those with limited treatment plans or no cure. The decision of going into clinical trials is one that should be made early in the disease while the victim still has the cognitive skills to determine if he or she is willing to take the risks. There is inherent risk in any new drug because it is just that—a new drug—and the potential side effects are not always fully known, especially in the early stages of the trials. Clinical trials are an extremely important part of finding improved therapies or a cure—but not necessarily for the person in the trial and most likely not today.

The research that is done today is for the future victims of the disease. Clinical trials involve years of testing and evaluation before the drug is presented to the FDA for approval because of the seemingly endless testing and safety protocols that must be designed for each drug trial. And through all the testing, protocols, dosing, and the evaluation of the drug that is tested for years, it may work for your victim but may not work for enough victims or there may have been too many side effects for the FDA to approve it. So then it is back to the drawing board.

Obviously, there are two opinions when addressing the subject of entering cognitively challenged people into clinical trials. The main issue is an AD victim's diminished capacity. Do these victims truly understand what could happen with drug side effects, the procedures they must endure, and why new medical personnel are groping them, taking blood, and the like? Lynne and I did two trials at Georgetown. The whole experience was different from the typical routine of going to the doctor, running some tests, and waiting for results. I cannot speak for other clinical trial environments, but the staff at Georgetown was very patient and very professional.

The trials involved both Lynne and me, not just Lynne, the AD victim. One of the conditions of being accepted into most AD trials is the presence and availability of the primary caregiver, not just the patient. While clinical trials involve blood and fluid testing, the taking of vital signs, MRIs, and the like, someone has to report on the patient's reactions and possible side effects, as the patient may not be able to fully understand or remember what to report. Also remember that we are dealing with a memory disorder, so someone needs to be responsible for the at-home dosing or other procedures that are required for the trial. And we don't want the cognitively challenged patient driving either, do we?

Like everything else in life, there are upsides and downsides when dealing with clinical trials. The upside—other than the obvious benefit of helping someone other than yourself—is the free medical screening, and in some trials, you may be paid for your time and transportation expenses. In our two trials at Georgetown, both of us were treated to a brownbag lunch at every visit. The downside (again, depending on the trial) is that there can be a lot of blood draws, injections, lumbar punctures, and of course, the possibility of side effects—some minor and some to be very concerned about.

I will warn you, as the trial coordinator will also warn you, that if you are expecting a cure or improvement with your participation in any clinical trial, you may be sorely disappointed. The clinical trial that you are in may run for a number of years of dosing and data collection. Depending on how the trial is going, the drug may never see the light of day ever again. It takes years of testing, data gathering, and analysis before the next phase commences, and of course, everything that is learned from the trial has to go through the FDA for approval or rejection. The FDA is, in fact, the ultimate government agency. It runs on reams of paper, miles of red tape, and a large population of bureaucrats. The bottom line is this—don't hold your breath waiting for a cure. The cure can be down the road a long distance from where you sit in today's clinical trial.

For each drug being tested, there are typically a minimum of three phases of trials. Phase I trials have a small patient population and are the first real step in the human part of the trials. Essentially, the drug has been proven safe in animals and is being tested on the human subjects. Phase II has a larger patient population, the bugs in the protocols have been worked out, and the dosing amounts have been established based on the lessons learned in Phase I testing.

Once the drug reaches Phase III testing, the drug is not on easy street, on its way to the FDA for approval. When a drug is in Phase III testing, there is an increased patient population, problems found in the prior testing have been ironed out, and the protocols have been adjusted accordingly. Basically, the drug worked safely in enough people in Phase II. There can still be possible side effects and other changes to the protocols and dosing since you are dealing with a much larger patient population and there is a much higher possibility of unforeseen events.

Our first trial was a Phase II intravenous drug that Lynne tolerated quite well, but it did come with a side effect. Throughout the trial, while she was receiving what was possibly the test medication versus the placebo, she gained weight every week. I told the trial coordinator, "You may not have found a cure for Alzheimer's, but you have found a cure for skinny." From the time that Lynne no longer received the intravenous dosing, she did not gain another pound.

This brings me to one of the usual conditions of participating in clinical trials. They request that you change as little as possible in your diet, exercise, and daily routine as possible. It is especially important for you or the victim's doctor to talk with the trial coordinator before adding, changing, or stopping any medications—whether AD-related or not, whether prescription or over-the-counter—because medication changes could have an effect on or interaction with the drug being tested. The possibility of Lynne gaining weight because of a change in diet or exercise was not possible since we followed the rules set forth in the testing protocol.

Our second trial was a Phase III oral medication that Lynne tolerated well, but because of a side effect, we subsequently had to drop out of this trial. Her side effect was an increased desire to urinate, which was one of the possible side effects that had been noted by the drug manufacturer.

With regard to the possible side effects of a trial drug, the trial coordinator, while aware of the previously reported side effects, will not tell you what to expect so that your victim won't develop or ignore any possible side effects. After all, the one of the purposes of the clinical trial is to determine all of the side effects, no matter their severity. And your victim may be the only trial participant with that side effect or the only one who showed no side effects at all. Also, the trial measures the placebo versus test drug versus the amount of the drug being administered. The trial coordinator cannot tell you anything about that either.

I had some limited knowledge of the clinical trial world from the business side. One of the clients Lynne and I had when we were operating the small-business support office was a doctor who assisted companies in the FDA approval process for new drugs and medical devices. This is where I learned that some of the reported side effects can be extremely rare at best. My favorite example is a clinical trial for an anti-gas medication; one of the side effects listed for presentation to the FDA for the drug's approval was suicide. Certainly flatulence, no matter how bad, does not rate suicide, at least in my mind. But because of FDA regulations, this "side effect" had to be listed since a trial participant had taken his own life during the course of the trial.

As a caregiver, I contribute to the AD and caregiver research world when and where I can. I have personally participated in a few studies, and while they are not as important as clinical trials, somebody valued my opinion and the opinions of others concerning caregiving efforts.

I received a survey from a Midwest university doing a study regarding caregiving of Alzheimer's patients. In the instructions, they estimated this survey would take about thirty minutes to complete. But that's one half hour in the real world.

While it actually took me about twenty minutes to mark the boxes and fill in the blanks, it, in fact, took over nine hours from beginning to end. As a caregiver, I learned how to prioritize early on. Completing this caregiving survey certainly did not take precedence over my usual duties. In those nine hours, I prepared and fed two meals, did two loads of laundry, had an hour-long visit with the hospice social worker, took four telephone calls, made no less than eight potty runs, put Lynne to bed twice, and managed to watch a few minutes of news while dinner was cooking. But I help out where I can.

Stories from the Real World

I have regaled you with stories of what daily life was like in our pre-Alzheimer's world and the nightmare that enveloped us when Lynne and my mother became part of the 5.4 million. Now I hope to give you a few more ideas on how to proceed, give you things to watch for, or just show you what you are doing is okay. That you really have not done anything wrong, contrary to what you may think or what others are telling you.

Just so you know going in; not all of these random stories are about my mother, my wife, or me, but they are good examples of some of the elements of caregiving that can make this job more than a little interesting. This job of caregiver is definitely not dull or for the faint of heart or weak of back or spirit.

We went to a national hardware chain store one day. I had started calling our outings "have wheelchair, will travel." Since I have shopped at most of the stores that we now frequent many times over the years, I have a good idea which stores to shop at when they are least likely to be busy.

My general appearance has gotten people's attention in the past. I am; some would say, an imposing figure at six foot six and 260 pounds. People have always tended to notice me. Now add a wheelchair-bound or slowly walking five-foot-two wife, and we are nearly impossible to miss. Picture my ailing wife, sitting hunched over in her wheelchair, a loaded cart, and a frenzied caregiver racing through the store, trying to grab up everything from a list of many projects to come, time permitting.

As we were heading for the checkout, two men passed going the opposite direction. One stopped and asked if I needed assistance with the cart, since I was pushing Lynne's wheelchair with one hand and pulling the cart behind me with the other. I smiled and thanked him for his kindness but told him I was okay and I would not need any assistance, as we were just a few feet from the checkout and would then be leaving.

While I was loading the merchandise into our truck, the two gentlemen we encountered at the checkout were heading for the parking lot. I again smiled and thanked the man for his offer of assistance. As I continued unloading the cart and prepared to put Lynne's wheelchair into the truck, the men lingered. The man who offered assistance in the store started chatting. He asked very sheepishly what was wrong with Lynne. I was quick to tell him she suffered from Early Onset Alzheimer's disease.

We talked for a few moments about caregiving, Alzheimer's disease, the bleak future, and my level of commitment to my wife and her care. As he was leaving, he offered his hand, smiled, and said, "I feel blessed having talked with you today. With all you have to do, your positive attitude, and your obvious love and caring manner in such difficult times, you can still smile and take time for others."

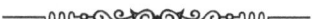

When Lynne and I were out and about in the middle stages of her disease, she would usually need to use the bathroom. With her vision problems, she needed assistance in most public restrooms, and I was the assistant. I always tried to plan our outings so that we would be near an AD victim- and caregiver-friendly bathroom. Since I knew her bathroom habits well, I could schedule and plan accordingly. Basically, I made sure that we were situated at the not-so-busy pet store and not the crowded department store at the right time.

At first, I always chose the ladies room for some reason. I tried to wait until the room was vacant. If we were joined "midstream," I would announce my presence to give ample warning to the unsuspecting. I seldom got more of a reaction than "Thanks for the warning," "No problem," or "I'll wait till you're done."

One day, the men's room was the only option, and it was vacant. We went in; she did her thing, and we were just reaching the door when a young man walked in. When he realized we were not two guys—and it was fairly obvious since Lynne was wearing a low-cut, very girlie blouse—he did a double take followed by another double take. We let him pass, and as we were leaving, I saw him sort of shake his head.

A few weeks later, I decided we would use the men's room again. This reaction was better—almost a funniest home video moment. A man came in, saw Lynne, excused himself for being in the ladies' room, and left. A moment later, he returned, again excused himself for being in the wrong bathroom, and started to leave. Before he got too far, I didn't have the heart to have him to go out and come back in again for fear he might actually end up in the ladies' room. I don't think he ever saw me, even though I was standing right beside Lynne, helping her dry her hands. He saw her, fixated on her, and reacted. And yes, she once again was wearing something low-cut and very girlie.

The reaction from the different bathrooms was not what I expected, but at the same time, I was not surprised. My presence in the ladies' room, helping my wife, appeared to be quite normal and unobtrusive to the other users of the facility. Lynne's presence in the men's room often made them obviously uncomfortable, dazed, and confused. It was like we had invaded the inner sanctum, violating some law of nature. The reactions were almost always the same. Women, who are more often the primary caregivers, accept me as the caregiver for a woman. Since fewer men are involved in the daily activities of adult care, they tend to be more easily embarrassed or surprised when an adult female is in the men's room, especially when she is dressed in very adult, feminine clothing.

The key to the story was to get Lynne to the bathroom, but the rest of the story falls in the category of having a bit of fun at someone else's expense. This is not exactly an indictment of shortsightedness or narrow-minded thinking but rather something fun to do just to gauge the reaction of strangers and how uncomfortable some can be.

———————

After Nichole and James had been together for a time, they fell in love and decided to be married. When Nichole told us of her pending nuptials, she had few details except for the fact that they were to be married the next summer. Since they had just become engaged, we were not surprised that the date had not been set. We figured that with James being in the Navy and knowing military red tape, the date would be set based on military schedule and church availability. At the time, Nichole was an elementary school teacher, so we assumed the wedding would be during the summer break.

Even though Lynne had shown some cognitive loss, we expected that Nichole would have included her mother in at least some aspects of the wedding planning. Lynne would have likely turned down an invitation to go mall-crawling or hopping from bridal shop to bridal shop. It would have been difficult for her to keep up with Nichole. But Lynne was hoping to be of some help to Nichole while she was planning the wedding.

A few days after the engagement had been announced, Nichole e-mailed us a picture of the wedding dress she had selected. She called a few hours later to get our opinion on the dress that she had already bought. It would have been nice if she had at least gone through the motions by sending Lynne a few options, even though she had already purchased the dress. Lynne's input would have been of no value to

Nichole, but it would have made Lynne feel like she was being included in the wedding preparation and her daughter's life.

It was never our desire to be included in the wedding or deeply involved in the preparation beyond just offering advice, opinions, and monetary assistance if needed. But the lack of communication from Nichole became so obvious that we only found out a few details when we received our wedding invitation in the mail. It was then that we were informed of the wedding date and location as well as the location of the wedding reception.

After seeing Lynne's obviously heartbroken reaction to receiving the invitation in the mail, a few days later, I asked whether she still wanted to attend the wedding. I told her to think seriously about it and make a decision and offered no opinion. When she made that decision, I asked her to tell me what decided and why. About three days passed, and she asked me for the details of the wedding. Aside from the date, time, and location and what I assumed the bride would be wearing, I had no other information. I supplied her with what I knew, and she continued to consider whether we would attend.

One of Lynne's concerns was at most of the weddings we had attended in the past, including Nichole's first wedding; I was the wedding photographer. Lynne was concerned that I would be shooting the wedding, and she would be left alone in an unfamiliar location among people she did not know.

I answered her questions about the wedding as best I could and assured her that I was not asked to shoot the wedding, so she would not be left alone at any time. Also, we would not be attending the reception, since she was very sensitive to noise and was becoming quite uneasy in crowds. With that, she continued to consider whether we would attend. I made it abundantly clear throughout her deliberation that it was totally her choice—that I was not rendering an opinion or making the decision for her. But her decision would have to be made in time for James to put us on the security list, since the wedding was to take place on base. We also had to go shopping for a wedding-appropriate dress for Lynne.

After several days of consideration and asking questions to verify what she thought she remembered and understood, Lynne decided that she did not want to attend. I told her I was okay with that if she was absolutely sure, but I needed to know, in case someone asked her reason for not wanting to attend Nichole's wedding. Lynne said without hesitation, "I don't feel like she wants me there."

If Nichole had made even a superficial effort to include Lynne and help me to allay Lynne's fears, I probably would have been able to convince Lynne that it would have been okay for us to attend. Sadly, it did not seem to matter to Nichole that her mother and I would not be attending her wedding.

It was important for Lynne to voice her opinion on two things, since she obviously had been hurt by Nichole's total exclusion concerning the wedding. Lynne felt bad about finally getting the few details of the wedding through the mail like everybody else, since Nichole could not find the time to call or visit to tell us anything about the wedding after she had bought the dress. It was also obvious that Nichole was making no effort to ensure her mother's comfort. Nichole should have considered Lynne's uneasiness when going to strange places, being around strangers, and the possibility of our becoming separated at the wedding.

So what's the purpose of this story? Disappointment is lurking around every corner. As I have said many times, keep your expectations low, and be prepared for disappointment. Above all else, be ready for others to do the disappointing for you, leaving you to clean up the mess that someone else has left behind. Others know that it's your job as the caregiver to clean up the mess, and they do not have to give a second thought to your victim's feelings or yours.

To add insult to injury, in the years since the wedding, Lynne and I have seen exactly one picture from the wedding that was shot with a cell phone. What makes it even sadder is that Lynne will never be able to see any photograph of the wedding that she chose not to attend because she was made to feel like damaged goods and an outsider to her daughter's life.

—⁓⁓⁓⁓⁓⁓⁓⁓⁓—

One day, Lynne got a call from our cell phone service provider. I naturally answered the telephone, since she was normally unable to find the telephone. "May I speak with Lynne Tutor?" My response, as it always was to whoever called asking for Lynne directly, was, "She is very sick and can't come to the telephone right now. I'm her husband: is there something I can help you with?"

The representative answered, "No, I'll call back some other time." As promised, she or another customer service representative called back multiple times. Each time, I would say my well-rehearsed lines and the representatives would say theirs. Once or twice a week for several weeks, the telephone would dutifully ring in the late afternoon. After several weeks, I would ask or demand they talk with me because Lynne was very sick and unable to talk on the telephone, and I would end up talking with them anyway. Their response was always, "We have to talk with her because the account is in her name."

After several attempts on my part and as many refusals on theirs, I finally had enough customer service contact. When the usual call came in one day, I had about as much as I could stand of being disturbed by our cell service provider. "May I speak with Lynne Tutor?" My response, which I had not practiced or even thought of before that moment, "I'm sorry, she has Alzheimer's disease right now. Would you like to talk to me or wait for a cure?"

After a short and obviously uncomfortable pause, I was told about upgrades to our service. I thanked her for the information that was so long in coming. She thanked me for my time, apologized for the disruptions, and wished us good luck.

I was sitting in the waiting area at our pharmacy, waiting for a new prescription of mine to be filled. I overheard the woman sitting with me while she was talking on her cell phone about waiting for her father's AD medication refill. After the call, since I am not the shy type when I hear of AD, I struck up a conversation about, of all things, Alzheimer's. We swapped a few caregiving stories over the next few minutes. I have told our story so many times; I have a capsule version down pat—wife and best friend with AD, solo caregiver, too many things to do, too little sleep, and no help in sight. You know the drill.

She assumed I was also waiting for AD medications. Not this time, I told her; this trip was for me. I told her I had recently been to the doctor and had an EKG run, and since my results came back okay, the doctor had decided which medication I needed. I told her I didn't trust the EKG results because it didn't show that I was suffering from a broken heart. Of course, I was kidding, but she started tearing up. With her voice cracking, she said, "You must really love her." The pharmacy tech called my name, and I said a quick good-bye, wished her luck, and beat a hasty retreat, hoping to avoid her tears.

A census worker called, inquiring about my mother. We spoke for about fifteen minutes about my mother and her temporary residence at Happy Valley. As we talked, I told her about Lynne, my care for her, and my devotion to the task of caring for my wife but also visiting my mother for a few hours every day. By the end of the conversation, she was not only praying for us, but also sobbing. I can have that kind of effect on people. The love I have for Lynne and the passion for and dedication to my job cannot be hidden, and I do not want it to be.

A mother was driving to the Minneapolis—St. Paul airport to pick up her daughter, who was returning from a business trip. The mother had driven this route a number of times before. Sadly, they found the mother, an AD victim, some six hundred miles from the Minneapolis—St. Paul area. She had gotten lost and apparently drove until she could find a familiar landmark. She had died from exposure, having left her car to find help when the car ran out of gas in northeast Wyoming. Had she not stopped along the way and used her credit card to buy gas, she likely would have been missing for far longer.

A woman in North Carolina who had dementia-related issues for some time still had the car keys and was often left home alone during the day. She had problems remembering where she was going, and on occasion drove past her destinations, including her own home. This apparently was not noticed by her husband, as he did not take away her car keys or have someone stay with her when he was not available. One day she left the house, driving the car. A search team found her abandoned car the next morning on a farm road not far from where she lived. Several months later, they found her body in the woods, where she had died of exposure.

A family in Wisconsin received a call from a sheriff's office in Florida, informing the family that a builder had unearthed the remains of the wife's father, who had disappeared from an Alzheimer's facility. It seems that he had wandered from the facility more than twenty years prior and had never been found.

Alzheimer's victim "Kate" was living with her daughter's family in an upscale suburban neighborhood. Kate had a history of escaping when left alone for more than a moment. One afternoon, Kate's daughter returned from the laundry room to Kate's previous location. After a search of the house and calls to the neighbors, Kate's daughter called the police to join in the frantic search of the neighborhood by family members and neighbors. As dusk was settling in, after a few hours of unsuccessful searching by neighbors, church members, and the police—including the police helicopter, it looked as if Kate was in real danger, but because of the approaching darkness, the search would have to wait until the next morning.

As the volunteers departed, one was taking out the bags of trash generated by the searchers. As the volunteer was stuffing the bags of trash into the garbage cans, a small "Help me" was heard over the rustle of trash bags.

Kate was still on the property. She had left the house and ended up between the garden shed and the decorative shrubbery behind the outbuilding. While the searchers had searched the house and the very large yard, nobody looked between the building and the shrubs.

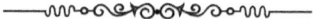

About eight months after my mother passed, I went to the bank to close out her checking and money market accounts. All of the checks had long cleared, and all direct deposits had stopped. There was no longer any reason to maintain her accounts since eventually the dreaded service charges would begin. This bank is one of the biggies, so service charges, maintenance fees, or some type of expense for these inactive accounts was inevitable.

Both of her accounts were interest-bearing accounts. They were not earning much interest, since the balances were just high enough to avoid the service fees. When I went to close the accounts, the assistant branch manager filled out the paperwork after quizzing the computer for the balance on both accounts. I learned a few days after the accounts were closed that he had added thirty cents to the existing balance on one of the accounts.

With the thirty cents the assistant manager added to the amount transferred into my account, I believe he single-handedly brought the big, big bank to its knees. My oversight and the manager's generosity caused an overdraft fee on the closed account because the amount withdrawn from the account was thirty cents higher than the balance. And this was just the beginning of all the chaos.

I called customer service to have them waive the overdraft fee after explaining my understanding of the situation and authorized them to take back their thirty cents from my account. It sounds simple enough for this big, big bank to move a lousy thirty cents from my account into their vault. Wrong! To make a very long and ridiculous story short, after six telephone calls back and forth with the big, big bank and spending God knows how much money in corporate man hours, paper, and computer time, they finally took their thirty cents back nearly three months after they gave it to me.

———∿◦◦ᡆᠧᠣᡬᡅᠥᠥᠬᢇ———

Lynne's story almost came to an end on 9/11. She was not at the Pentagon, but she was within sight of the Pentagon. (A few years prior to the attack, she frequently attended meetings in that part of the building.) During the ordeal of 9/11, I spoke with Lynne before and after the plane struck the Pentagon, which was just over a mile from where she was working.

After the attack, the federal government offices in the Washington metropolitan area were all ordered to evacuate. At the time, Lynne was working at the FDIC in Arlington, Virginia. When the evacuation order was given, Lynne, along with everyone else, left the building, and most of the people awaiting rides were standing in the sheltered area at the end of the building.

In our previous conversation, I told her that I would pick her up at this sheltered area, feeling confident that, in the panic, the cell service would be overloaded. So after flying down Route 66 from Fairfax into Arlington without any cell service, as I predicted, I knew where Lynne would be waiting. I also had given her a second and third pick-up location should they have to leave the FDIC grounds. I like being prepared.

My trip to Arlington was much faster than usual, as I was driving a late-model Suburban with a paint scheme similar to the Virginia State Police cars. Add to that flashing headlights and not being afraid to drive at a high rate of speed on the shoulder like the police who had passed us trying to get to the Pentagon as fast as possible.

Once I made the turn onto the street where the sheltered area was located, it took me no time to find Lynne. It seems that my always-inquisitive little wife was standing in the middle of the street, watching the black smoke rising from the Pentagon. Had I not been quicker on the brakes, I surely would have hit her at a high rate of speed and likely would have ended her story on 9/11.

Our escape from Arlington back to Fairfax was far less eventful. It seems that everybody who drove to work that day was released simultaneously, so the roads were filled. But it did not take us the three hours to drive the normally thirty-minute trip. Having lived in the Washington suburbs all of my life and having worked as an ice cream vendor during college through nearly every subdivision in Arlington and Fairfax, I knew every back road and cut-through. I got us home in a fraction of the time that most everybody else had to endure.

One day, I was keeping my idle hands busy by cleaning out the gutters and downspouts, preparing for a hurricane. Armed with the bed monitor, I was cleaning out the gutters around the house when, of all things, we had an earthquake. For people who live in places like California, earthquakes are commonplace, but here in Northern Virginia, the closest we have to an earthquake is the occasional tremor that most people would not know about unless they saw it on the news.

On this particular day, there was a 5.8 earthquake some sixty miles southwest of our home while I was about ten feet up the ladder. After the shaking of both the ladder and its owner subsided, I went in to check on Lynne, who felt the shaking but was not really aware of what was going on. The next day, after I felt confident (or at least hopeful) we were not going to be shaken again; I continued cleaning the gutters for the hurricane that turned out to be little more than a breezy, rainy day.

A few days later, Tropical Storm Lee dumped several inches of rain on us over a short period of time, causing flooding across our backyard. Because of all the debris that had stuck in our fence and because I did not want to lose the fence, I donned my rain gear and went out in a hurricane-quality rainstorm to remove all the debris from our fence in three feet of rushing water. After being in the onslaught and flooding, I did save the fence and returned to the house drenched from top to toe. The bottom line is that while caregiving is a full-time job, sometimes you have to find part-time work to keep you distracted, keep a roof over your head, or keep your basement dry.

———∿∿∞ᘓᖶᓂᖶᘏᘏ∿∿———

For quite some time after Lynne was no longer able to work, she was still able to go for her long walks around the neighborhood every day. Every morning after rush hour, she would leave the house and go on her established route, which she had walked hundreds of times. I knew how long it would take her to navigate the several blocks, allowing for occasional stops to chat with people along the way and to pet the various dogs she came across.

One day, I looked out my office window, waiting for her to make her customary appearance to walk the last four hundred feet of her route. I spotted Lynne and a gentleman walking down the street being followed by a construction vehicle. I ran out the front door and met them partway. The man told me that she had appeared to be a little confused, so he used her medical alert necklace to get her information. He walked her home instead of calling me to come pick her up. The moral of the story should be fairly obvious, and maybe you have heard it before—be prepared for what is never going to happen, because it probably will.

Lynne had gotten confused after she stopped to watch some people working at a construction site about two blocks from home. She stopped to watch the proceedings, and when she had seen enough, she started walking the wrong direction because the construction vehicles parked on the side of the road had blocked the familiar landmarks. Fortunately, the site foreman recognized Lynne's confusion and spotted the medical alert necklace. A potential disaster was averted.

Near the end of Lynne's morning walks, if I felt she was not at her best, I would follow her along the route to make sure she was turning at the right places and not putting herself in dangerous situations. If I had to stop her along the way, I would always tell her I wanted her to come with me while I ran an errand so she would not suspect I was following her, not trusting her to be safe on her walks.

Lynne continued to walk for a few more months until we felt she had too many problems remembering the turning points on her route. But we decided when it was time to stop the morning walks. It was not just my decision; it was ours. Remember sick, not stupid.

Many Lessons Learned

Caregiving is all about learning and then applying your newfound education. I am no different from any other caregiver. It took time and errors for me to evolve from novice to capable.

- Patience is the first thing I learned. Patience is a thing that you have to learn over and over, as the stress of an ever-changing situation destroys what little normalcy you experience when caring for a terminally ill loved one.
- Remember, no matter how hard you push, Alzheimer's will push back, and it pushes harder than you can. Ultimately, it will win the war and most of the battles.
- Time is something you never have enough of and will never get back again. Plan to the best of your ability.
- When developing plans, keep your expectations low, and then build on your success if you can. Plans always have to be changed—usually not for the better and always for all the wrong reasons.

Strangely enough, when my father passed away, even though my mother was super organized, a formidable force, and always the go-to, get-it-done analyst at the Pentagon, she was no more prepared for my father's death after having six months' warning than if he had dropped dead on the street. There was no will, other than a few notes there were no funeral arrangements, and truly no direction on what needed to be done following my father's passing except for going back to work and trying recover from the pain she had endured.

Denial of the final outcome only makes things worse. I swore that I would not do the same thing if the situation ever presented itself. Keeping the truth hidden from someone who is going to die does nothing more than make a bad situation more difficult and ultimately impossible for all concerned. I think the situation that my mother went through only provided me with the strength to deal with the prognosis of both my mother and my wife. And whether Lynne goes in months or years, I have everything ready, so the burden of what happens next is no longer a burden to me or anyone else should something happen to me first.

Have my mother, Lynne, and I been sent on a mission from God to be in this war that, currently and most likely for the foreseeable future, has millions of victims without as much as in inkling of what causes the disease, how to cure it, how to develop more effective treatments, or a way to prevent it? Even if we were not tasked for this mission, maybe our participation—especially Lynne's—will be one of the keys to a future without Alzheimer's.

Having seen firsthand and heard stories from other caregivers, as well as healthcare professionals, I firmly believe the healthcare system is not able to work with Alzheimer's patients and their families. Alzheimer's takes away the patient's ability to communicate effectively, so emergent problems that could be handled with simple communication become major problems without effective communication.

I can understand doctors not feeling the need to send you out with information regarding a fatal disease. After all, you or your loved one may have just received the news of a pending loss of life, but your doctor is losing a patient, which will affect the practice's bottom line. I am not saying all doctors are totally absorbed with concerns about money. I have seen many who are truly concerned—not only with the patient and their care, but also with the family.

Now with all these nasty words about the money-grubbing doctors and their lack of caring and understanding aside, there are a few good guys out in the real world. The neurologist with the big mustache who finally diagnosed Lynne understood our dwindling bank account as well as our growing frustration at not finding a diagnosis. He was kind enough to provide all of his services at no charge even after Lynne had qualified for Medicare.

I look back at the struggles we went though in trying to find a reason for Lynne's initial problems—the fruitless search that cost years of treatment time and many thousands of dollars. I should have pushed the very arrogant second neurology practice to run more tests. I just did not have enough knowledge to force the issue. On our initial visit, I told them to do whatever was necessary and run any tests, no matter what the cost. We had to find out what was wrong with Lynne. But in their less-than-eager approach to do more than the bare minimum, they did not run all the available tests. Had they done the job right, the result still would have come up as Alzheimer's, but Lynne could have been on medication three years sooner and possibly could have had a little more quality time.

To add insult to injury, when Lynne applied for Social Security Disability benefits, this practice wanted her to make a return visit as a follow-up prior to them releasing her information to SSA. In my conversation with the practice concerning the follow-up request, I was "erroneously" told (a diplomatic way to say being lied to) that it was SSA procedure for the practice to do a follow-up examination so they could complete the required forms and determine what Lynne's current condition was as compared to her previous visits, of which there were many. I knew this was erroneous, as I read the rules on

SSA disability procedures in granting benefits. So when this follow-up request was made, it raised a red flag, and I called "Abby," Lynne's SSA point of contact, to verify my understanding.

When I called the neurology practice a second time concerning the need for a follow-up visit to clarify their understanding of the rules, I was told that unless we came in for the follow-up visit at our cost, the practice would not release the information to SSA, thus jeopardizing Lynne's claim. This was an idle threat (or thinly veiled blackmail), as I had spoken with Abby concerning this follow-up question. Abby indicated that we could proceed without the file from this practice without any risk of jeopardizing Lynne's case. Again, we received some erroneous information from this doctor's office.

For the uninitiated, SSA selects medical professionals to examine the applicant and render opinions on the applicant's illness or condition. It is not the responsibility of a previous doctor to perform follow-up examinations for SSA. It is the previous doctor's responsibility to send the requested documentation so SSA can determine the applicant's eligibility for benefits, not to keep milking the cash cow. I also assumed that, if after more than a dozen office visits and all the tests they had performed, since they did not find the answer before, there wasn't much hope that they would find the solution with a follow-up.

So what have we learned? No matter how good the doctor is (or thinks he or she is), they are not above the rules, no matter how many rules the doctors make up for themselves. This practice had made a lot of money off Lynne, and they were banking on our not knowing the rules so they could make more money off of her. For the uninitiated, SSA medical examinations for disability claims are at no charge to the applicant. Of the three doctors to whom SSA sent Lynne for second opinions, two of them provided the most in-depth exams we had seen in our search for a diagnosis. These second opinions were not just rubber-stamping *denied* on the paperwork.

Lynne's disability award, on the first attempt, was not based on her Alzheimer's disease, since she had not been diagnosed at that point. Her disability award was based on loss of visual acuity.

In order to make the AD caregiving lifestyle work in the non-AD world, there needs to be a type of registry for Alzheimer's victims and their primary caregivers. This resource could be used by state and local governments in times of emergency; they could contact families concerning programs and services, and my personal favorite, alert the DMV concerning a possible or probable AD patient continuing to drive. This registry could also be used in a commercial aspect by vendors specializing in the needs of AD patients and their caregivers to market products and services. Again, too much time is spent searching the Internet, making telephone calls, and driving around trying to find the tools of the trade needed when caring for anyone with a long-term or terminal disease.

You—Caregiver

If you are new to caregiving, the first step that you have probably already taken is to come to grips with the role that you are now assuming. You also have to help your Alzheimer's victim with his or her new role. Then the two of you have to decide when, how, and how much to tell your family and friends about the fact that your AD victim is just that—a terminally ill victim of Alzheimer's disease. Be prepared to answer questions, maybe dry a few tears, dispel misinformation about the disease, and start laying the ground work for what you and your AD victim expect to happen in the future. Focus on the level of support you will need from family and friends.

Before I get to the lecture, it is important that you understand the basics. You cannot take care of your loved one if you are sick or dead. This is a tough job that will take everything out of you—physically and emotionally. It is important for you to keep up with whatever health issues you have or may develop. But be aware of possible drug side effects before you start a new prescription. As the AD progresses and more victim support is required, it gets harder to maintain your health. So approach your health issues with the same aggression as you do your caregiving duties.

After years of sleep deprivation, tiredness or exhaustion become commonplace. And with that come sluggish responses, disorganized thinking, and the constant need to reschedule most non-caregiving activities. Tiredness leads to absolute exhaustion, which often leads to the possibility of making mistakes. This is where the years of caregiving experience, which hopefully has become more of an instinct, take over. This is when the smart play might be to call in the cavalry or turn to respite care at the local care facility. I just dig down deeper and carry on with my caregiving duties—just at a more measured and reduced pace when possible. And for those pesky chores around the house, I just prioritize and postpone as much as possible.

When you start taking over the adult personal responsibilities that we have all been doing for ourselves since childhood, you not only have to do these tasks while convincing and reassuring your AD loved one, but also keep from making the victim feel stupid, embarrassed, or like a child.

If your relationship included intimacy, remember to put it out of your mind while you are assisting the victim. Even though you may have had years of sex with the pre-AD person that person has likely changed mentally. So trying to be intimate may ruin the trust that you worked so hard to develop or maintain. To be brutally frank, having sex with a cognitively- or memory-challenged person could be viewed by the AD victim as rape or assault. My best advice is to keep it in your pants! (I know this is very sexist, but you get the idea.)

While I am on the subject of intimacy, if the opportunity presents itself for having sex with someone other than your partner, you know the person you are caring for; it is totally up to you how to proceed. I am still married to Lynne, and as long as she is still living, I do not feel that having sexual relations with another person is morally right. Even though to her, I am usually just someone who takes care of her, I know I am still her husband, and it would not be fair to cheat on her—even though the person who she has become, in her mind, has no emotional connection to me.

Use your own moral compass when making a decision like this, and remember, it's your face in the mirror. If you do find intimacy elsewhere, remember to leave your germs where you found them. Don't bring them home to infect your loved one. I know I sound a bit holier-than-thou, but put yourself in your loved one's shoes. When your loved one was healthy, would he or she have given you permission to go sleeping around? This is not a case of when the cat's away the mice will play. This is real life, not an opportunity to go out and get a little on the side. But it's up to you. I am not your conscience, parent, priest, or AD victim; it's your choice.

The role of caregiver—whether the patient is an adult or a child suffering from a temporary condition or a terminal disease—requires a commitment from you. You know that when caring for a terminally ill person that your level of commitment and the sacrifices that you have to make, the closer the end comes, can be even more potentially devastating to you even though you have been caring for the victim for years building up to the end.

I don't care what your previous life was like. Much of who you were before your loved one's diagnosis will be a distant memory for you and possibly a bone of contention between you, your AD loved one, and family members. In the early stages of the disease, life as you know it will remain much the same as it has in the recent years before the diagnosis. But as the disease increases its presence in both of your lives, gone will be the ten-hour workdays in the office, playing a quick round of golf or a few sets of tennis on the weekends, the daily jog, the three-day weekend vacations, and even simple things like going out and having a drink with your friends.

I cannot stress this enough—your life is going to be put on hold for the foreseeable future. If you are a solo caregiver, like I am, you will spend many hours longing for the good old days. I've been there, done that, and gotten over that—for the most part. I strongly recommend that to keep your head in the game, before you are forced into abandoning parts of your pre-AD life, start shedding activities early or at least start cutting back.

Do not waste your time fighting the disease; the disease will win every time. It will take your loved one and everything you hold dear; it does not care. That being said, other than the ADL responsibilities we all have to handle, what else can you do? Find a way to vent your frustrations, find a diversion that you can drop at a moment's notice, or go back to a hobby you may have given up in the past. I started researching the family tree on one of the very popular genealogy websites. It is perfect for us, because I am quiet and sit at a computer in the bedroom across the hall from where Lynne is sleeping. If she needs anything, I am just a few steps away from her bedside.

This section of my book is about you. By becoming the caregiver, whether solo or primary, you are making a commitment to your loved one that you will be there no matter how bad it gets. Trust me when I say that it will get bad, and bad will turn into worse. And then it really starts going downhill after that. If you can honestly say to yourself, *I can handle this,* without any reservation, knowing full well that there is absolutely no upside for you, then you are two things—a caregiver and a liar.

After your loved one enters the closing stages of this disease, take some time to look at them while they sleep. If you are not relieved by the quiet and peacefulness, then the next part of this will mean nothing. This is a preview of the actual final stage of any disease—of any life. For our purposes, let's call it stage eight of Alzheimer's disease. And you will certainly not need a psychic to look into this future; this is a preview of your loved one's death. You both have hopefully fought the good fight; you have done absolutely everything humanly possible for your loved one, but now your job is done.

Take a moment after this preview, and look back at the beginning— possibly even before the diagnosis—when the concept of caring for your loved one was a new, fresh idea. While you certainly were not looking forward to it, somewhere in the back of your mind, you were preparing yourself. You knew the disease would take away the personality of your loved one while giving you many new responsibilities.

I have often said that I would not wish this job or this disease on anybody. But even with some of the mistakes I made along the way and the heartache that I experience every day while taking care of Lynne, I never stopped loving her. I never lost sight of who she was, and I never failed to do my very best for her. What does this have to do with you? Call it a challenge from a very tired caregiver who hopefully has conveyed to you information, humor, and an increased desire to do for your loved one everything I did for mine without any regrets except regretting what could have been in the years that the disease took away.

Your goal, whether you volunteered for this job or not, is to do your absolute best. Never take your frustrations (of which there will be many) out on your loved one, and be prepared for the worst. Rejoice in little improvements wherever they can be found. They will most likely be short-lived and fleeting at best. When you see any improvements, do not misunderstand what these improvements are. It's not a cure. It's not remission, and it's not something you can hold on to. I saw these improvements in Lynne over the years. They were either a tease by the disease or a gift from God to help me remember who Lynne used to be and why I continue to do my best for her.

I do not know you, but I know you. And the person I know you to be will be in my position far too soon for absolutely the wrong reason. I pray for you and your loved one as you travel down this very rocky road to the end. I also pray for you, as I do for myself, that once our job is done; we can find our way back into a normal life. I don't know how that will happen since my best friend will not be there to help me reestablish a normal life. But I know that when she's gone, I will miss her terribly—but she will be in a far better place, free of her disease. And I will be more than okay with that.

My Closing, My Challenge

You may think, *Okay, Superman, if you're so busy twenty hours a day, caring for Lynne, taking care of the pets, working on the house, and doing everything else, where did you find the time to write the book?* Like I said, some of this epic is built around notes and e-mails that I gathered over the years, parts were written on scraps of paper while cooking dinner or doing other chores, and the balance was written while Lynne slept in the mornings. I even wrote a portion while sitting in the front yard on my lawn tractor.

Many have encouraged me to write this to help others. Call it a request from the people in the trenches and those who fear the possibility of AD trench warfare, call it therapy for a former writer who has always embraced the power of the pen, or call it part of my assignment from God to help not only my wife and my mother, but also caregivers and disease victims in the real world. I did not find the time; I made the time.

Our son-in-law, James, is justifiably concerned that Nichole may develop a neurologic condition since her grandmother had Parkinson's and her mother has Alzheimer's, or that some other debilitating illness may befall her. His biggest concern is whether he will be able to step up to the plate like I have. After all, according to many observers, I have set the bar extremely high for caregiving. My answer to James and others who have voiced the same concern is to turn to God for strength, courage, and guidance. Also, look inside yourself to see if you are willing to sacrifice to the level that other caregivers, no matter what the disease or condition, have had to sacrifice.

I often say that I would never wish any disease on anyone for any reason. But I sure wish a few folks could stand in my shoes for just a day. Hopefully they would gain an appreciation of the value of life, the true meaning of love, and the peace that comes with answering the call when someone needs you. I am not saying that, as a caregiver, I am any better than anybody else; I think it's fairly obvious. What separates me from many others is the fact that I will never give up.

People need to understand that it's not all about large bank accounts, big houses, expensive cars, the latest tech gadgets, or anything else that you can't take with you; it is about knowing what is important in life. Trust me when I say this; it all comes into sharp focus when the doctor says a word like *Alzheimer's*. And if you don't understand what's more important than money, property, and keeping up with the Joneses, you're reading this book for the humor—certainly, not for the caregiver information.

Someplace, there are answers to whether you will be able to rise to face the many challenges and stay the course for as long as it takes. But you cannot really find the answer before the question of whether you can be a caregiver ever comes up. I was able to ease into the role. Some have the caregiver role thrust upon them with a telephone call in the middle the night. It kind of makes you wish you paid more attention while reading this!

I am certainly not the best writer, but what I know is that when Lynne's time on this earth comes to an end and Alzheimer's has claimed yet another victim, these things will be true:

- I may not be the smartest guy around, but I certainly married well.
- I never put her in danger; I never raised a hand to her or my voice at her.
- I never placed my needs above hers.
- I did my best to never make her feel like less of a person, damaged goods, or stupid.

- I never let a day go by that I didn't try to find a better way to help her.
- I never cheated on her.
- I never failed to thank God for the skills and stamina I have needed to care for her.
- I never stopped loving her.
- I never gave up on my best friend and our friendship.

Resources and
Other Information

The Seven Stages of Alzheimer's

I nstead of reinventing the wheel, I borrowed the Alzheimer's Association's list of the seven stages of Alzheimer's from their website *(www.alz.org)*.

Alzheimer's symptoms vary. The stages below provide a general idea of how abilities change during the course of the disease. Remember, it is difficult to place a person with Alzheimer's in a specific stage, as stages may overlap.

Not everyone will experience the same symptoms or progress at the same rate. This seven-stage framework is based on a system developed by Barry Reisberg, MD, clinical director of the New York University School of Medicine's Silberstein Aging and Dementia Research Center.

Stage 1   No impairment (normal function)

The person does not experience any memory problems. An interview with a medical professional does not show any evident symptoms of dementia.

Stage 2   Very mild cognitive decline (may be normal age-related changes or earliest signs of Alzheimer's disease)

The person may feel as if he or she is having memory lapses—forgetting familiar words or the location of everyday objects. But no symptoms of dementia can be detected during a medical examination or by friends, family, or coworkers.

Stage 3 Mild cognitive decline (early-stage Alzheimer's can be diagnosed in some, but not all, individuals with these symptoms)

Friends, family, or coworkers begin to notice difficulties. During a detailed medical interview, doctors may be able to detect problems in memory or concentration. Common stage 3 difficulties include:

- noticeable problems coming up with the right word or name;
- trouble remembering names when introduced to new people;
- having noticeably greater difficulty performing tasks in social or work settings;
- forgetting material that one has just read;
- losing or misplacing a valuable object;
- increased trouble with planning or organizing.

Stage 4 Moderate cognitive decline (mild or early-stage Alzheimer's disease)

At this point, a careful medical interview should be able to detect clear-cut symptoms in several areas:

- forgetfulness of recent events;
- impaired ability to perform challenging mental arithmetic—for example, counting backward from one hundred by sevens;

- greater difficulty performing complex tasks, such as planning dinner for guests, paying bills, or managing finances;
- forgetfulness about one's own personal history;
- becoming moody or withdrawn, especially in socially or mentally challenging situations.

Stage 5   Moderately severe cognitive decline (moderate or mid-stage Alzheimer's disease)

Gaps in memory and thinking are noticeable, and individuals begin to need help with day-to-day activities. At this stage, those with Alzheimer's may:

- be unable to recall their own address or telephone number or the high school or college from which they graduated;
- become confused about where they are or what day it is;
- have trouble with less challenging mental arithmetic, such as counting backward from forty by subtracting fours or from twenty by twos;
- need help choosing proper clothing for the season or the occasion;
- still remember significant details about themselves and their family;
- still require no assistance with eating or using the toilet.

Stage 6 Severe cognitive decline (moderately severe or mid-stage Alzheimer's disease)

Memory continues to worsen, personality changes may take place, and individuals need extensive help with daily activities. At this stage, individuals may:

- lose awareness of recent experiences as well as of their surroundings;
- remember their own name but have difficulty with their personal history;
- distinguish familiar and unfamiliar faces but have trouble remembering the name of a spouse or caregiver;
- need help dressing properly and they, without supervision, make mistakes such as putting pajamas over daytime clothes or shoes on the wrong feet;
- experience major changes in sleep patterns— sleeping during the day and becoming restless at night;
- need help with the details of toileting (for example, flushing the toilet, wiping, or disposing of tissue properly);
- have increasingly frequent trouble controlling their bladder or bowels;
- experience major personality and behavior changes, including suspiciousness and delusions (such as believing that their caregiver is an imposter) or compulsive, repetitive behavior like hand-wringing or tissue shredding.
- Tend to wander or become lost

Stage 7 **Very severe cognitive decline (severe or late-stage Alzheimer's disease)**

In the final stage of this disease, individuals lose the ability to respond to their environment, to carry on a conversation, and eventually, to control movement. They may still say words or phrases.

At this stage, individuals need help with much of their daily personal care, including eating or using the toilet. They may also lose the ability to smile, to sit without support, and to hold up their heads. Reflexes become abnormal. Muscles grow rigid. Swallowing impaired.

Possible Signs of
Alzheimer's disease

I also borrowed the Alzheimer's Association's list of possible signs of Alzheimer's disease from their website *(www.alz.org)*.

- Memory loss that disrupts daily life—forgetting important dates, asking for the same information over and over, relying on memory aides.
- Challenges in planning or solving problems—losing the ability to develop and follow plans or work with numbers, trouble following a familiar recipe or keeping track of monthly bills, or difficulty in concentrating or taking much longer to do things than before.
- Difficulty completing familiar tasks—driving to familiar locations, managing a budget, or remembering the rules of a favorite game.
- Confusion with time or place—losing track of dates, seasons, or the passage of time. A person may forget where he or she is or how he or she got there.
- Trouble understanding visual images and spatial relationships—difficulty reading, judging distance, and determining color or contrast.
- New problems with words in speaking or writing—problems with following or joining conversation. A person may stop in the middle of conversation and have no idea how to continue or may repeat himself or herself. The individual may struggle

with vocabulary, have problems finding the right word, or call things by the wrong name.

- Misplacing things and losing the ability to retrace steps—putting things in strange places. A person may lose things, be unable to recall where he or she has been, or be unable to retrace his or her steps.
- Decreased or poor judgment. A person may use poor judgment when handling money. He or she may pay less attention to grooming or keeping clean.
- Withdrawal from work and social activities. A person may start to remove himself or herself from hobbies, social activities, or projects at work.
- Changes in mood and personality. A person may become confused, suspicious, depressed, fearful, or anxious. He or she may become easily upset when out of his or her comfort zone.

The Internet Resources

H ere are some of the websites I have found useful and always reliable. There are countless AD and caregiving websites and blogs. Treat each as information and not the gospel. Double check sites you feel may be beneficial before taking any action.

AD and Caregiver Information

The Alzheimer's Association	*alz.org*
Federal Government AD Site	*alzheimers.gov*
Medicare	*medicare.gov*
Elder Care Forum	*agingcare.com*
Caregiver Resources	*care.com*
Alzheimer's Daily News	*agelessdesign.com*
Alzheimer's and Dementia Weekly	*alzheimersweekly.com*
Resource/Blog	*alzheimersspeaks.com*
Caregiver Resources	*helpguide.org*
AD Information	*mayoclinic.com*

Equipment and Supplies

General	*alzstore.com*
	allegromedical.com
	spinlife.com
	medline.com
	amazon.com
	overstock.com
Vitamins and Nutrition	*vitacost.com*
Clinical Trials	*clinicaltrials.gov*
Senior Housing	*aplaceformom.com*

www.ingramcontent.com/pod-product-compliance
Lightning Source LLC
Chambersburg PA
CBHW061352280526
45784CB00001B/229